DR. JEN'S GUIDE TO BREASTFEEDING

Meet Your Breastfeeding Goals by Understanding
Your Body and Your Baby

By Dr. Jennifer Thomas, MD, MPH, IBCLC, FAAP, FABM

With Lisa Holewa

©Copyright 2012

Hale Publishing, L.P.

Dr. Jen's Guide To Breastfeeding

Meet Your Breastfeeding Goals by Understanding
Your Body and Your Baby

Dr. Jennifer Thomas, MD, MPH, IBCLC, FAAP, FABM
With Lisa Holewa
© Copyright 2012

Hale Publishing, L.P.
1712 N. Forest St.
Amarillo, TX 79106-7017
806-376-9900
800-378-1317

www.iBreastfeeding.com

Library of Congress Control Number: 2012936000
ISBN-13: 978-0-9847746-4-7

Printing and Binding: Edwards Brothers Malloy

Dedicated to Alex, Ryan, Ethan, and Upton. And written with gratitude to all the breastfeeding mothers and babies that I have met for their courage and inspiration, always reminding me how blessed I am to do what I do.

TABLE OF CONTENTS

INTRODUCTION

For one long, hot summer in high school, I worked at a shopping mall maternity store. A maternity store that, it turned out, was known for its extensive collection of nursing bras in sizes with bigger numbers and more letters than I'd ever seen together. And one of my jobs was to fit the customers with the proper bras.

My manager showed me exactly how to measure, what numbers to add, where to subtract. And yet, the first time I found myself in a fitting room with a customer who needed help, well, I can only say that nothing I'd seen in the girls' locker room had prepared me for *this*. Who knows where I put the measuring tape or whether I used any math or where I looked while trying to avoid looking at *anything*—I do know that I blurted out the biggest number and letter combination I could think of, grabbed a corresponding bra from the rack, and hustled the customer toward the cash register.

Sadly, it turned out that the biggest size I could think of wasn't that big, here in the nursing bra world. And my manager could tell with a glance that I wasn't even in the ballpark. I spent much of the rest of that summer sorting hangers in the stock room.

Oddly enough, I completely blocked this incident from memory for many years, more than a dozen, until the morning of April 14, 1999. I was in the hospital with my newborn daughter, beautiful and perfect and oh-so-lovely...and red-faced and screaming, still unable to attach herself to my nipple to begin this beautiful mother-daughter breastfeeding dance. And so we hurried down the hallway to a classroom, where a half-dozen other screaming babies and exhausted new moms listened to a very young woman with colorful scrubs and a Scooby Doo voice use a baby doll and handheld cloth nipple to demonstrate how to "pop the baby on" to achieve a proper latch.

"Rou just ROP the raby on," she said repeatedly with her Scooby-enthusiasm, madly flopping the floppy doll onto the useless nipple. I watched and listened intently, desperately, my day-old daughter crying at my shoulder. I needed this to make sense. And out of nowhere this image popped into my head, this memory of me trying to rush a needy nursing mom out the door with a bra that would maybe, if stretchy, cover one breast.

And I knew, for certain, this would not be easy.

I first met Jenny Thomas in college when we were randomly assigned to be freshman roommates. She was in the university's pre-medical scholars program. I was in the journalism school. We both grew up in the Midwest; our parents both had three children each about the same ages apart, but that and our dorm room were perhaps all that we shared. Still, we became great friends. Her parents were what were referred to as "health nuts" when we grew up in the 1970s and 80s, mostly vegetarian, marathon runners who cared deeply about good nutrition and exercise. I can still hear the bitterness in Jenny's voice as she recounted being the only child at school forced to bring little sandwich bags filled with matchstick cut carrot sticks on outings to McDonald's, munching those while her friends ate hamburgers and French fries.

Years later when Jenny was studying to be a doctor and pregnant with her first son, it was her "granola" mother's voice and example that inspired her to breastfeed—she had been breastfed, and so she would breastfeed her child. Her life at the time was overwhelming; she was a medical resident studying to be a pediatrician, working impossibly long hours—there would be no such thing for her as maternity leave or pumping breaks or sympathetic bosses. But, following her mother's example, she simply assumed breastfeeding would work, naturally.

Interestingly, though she was studying to be a baby doctor, Jenny had learned nothing in medical school about the benefits of breastfeeding. That's correct—nothing. This was during the 1990s—the "Breast is Best" campaign was already part of our nation's culture; the U.S. government had established breastfeeding goals as part of its Healthy People 2000 initiative; the American Academy of Pediatrics (AAP) had been officially recommending breastfeeding over bottlefeeding for more than a decade. Yet, as an aspiring baby doctor, Jenny had taken part in classroom "taste tests" of leading infant formulas. She could recite formula ingredient lists, noting the percentage and purpose of each additive. But she never encountered a nursing mother until she was a medical resident and accidentally walked into a new mom's hospital room while the woman was breastfeeding. Embarrassed and uncertain what to do, she turned and walked from the room.

And so, as an overwhelmed new mom, her enthusiasm for breastfeeding already waning and her exhaustion rising, she felt a sense of relief and a bit of giddy happiness as she watched the cases of free formula arrive on her doorstep, courtesy of eager formula representatives. Jenny nursed her first son for exactly six weeks.

Interestingly, Dr. Jen is not the only pediatrician in our country who didn't learn much in medical school about breastfeeding. New moms may look to their babies' pediatricians for support and guidance during those difficult first weeks and months of nursing. And yet, a recent survey of pediatricians showed that 40 percent of those responding *did not* feel knowledgeable about breastfeeding. More telling, only 65 percent of pediatricians responding to a 2004 AAP survey reported receiving *any* education about breastfeeding while in medical school or during residency. Thankfully, this is changing. But what impact does this lack of medical education have when a new breastfeeding mom worries at her child's two-week checkup that he seems colicky, or is concerned about whether she is producing enough milk, or notes that her infant gags or fusses while nursing? Can well-intentioned, but poorly-trained baby doctors actually help derail a new mother's breastfeeding efforts?

Dr. Jen first began thinking about these questions a few years after her own breastfeeding attempts, when she attended a medical conference and sat in on a seminar about breastfeeding. As she listened to the speaker outline the scientific research about the remarkable medical benefits of breastmilk, she thought: *Why didn't I ever learn this in medical school?*

And so Dr. Jen's natural sense of competitiveness (*Why does she know all this cool stuff and I don't?*) joined with her own personal breastfeeding experience, compelling her to learn more. With a dawning awareness of the deep void faced by nursing mothers in need of support—and its ultimate effect on her youngest, most vulnerable patients—she became one of a handful of pediatricians who are also board-certified lactation consultants.

Dr. Jen now holds all sorts of titles related to her expertise on all matters related to breastfeeding. She speaks regularly at national breastfeeding conventions, educating physicians about breastfeeding, talking about how pediatricians can integrate breastfeeding guidance into their practices, and presenting seminars about how to use the latest medical research to achieve breastfeeding success.

But perhaps even more important, she is a practicing pediatrician who encounters new moms every day in her practice who are struggling with breastfeeding. She is the mother of three children. She nursed all of her boys—her two younger sons well into toddlerhood. And she knows that women struggling with breastfeeding need a little bit more than advice and reassurance—sometimes, they actually need a plan.

This book provides that plan, coupled with real medical information (the geek kind, for those who are into that kind of stuff!), guidance, and reassurance. And perhaps more important, it empowers moms with the knowledge they need to trust their instincts and their bodies to feed their babies.

— *Lisa Holewa*

PART 1.
DR. JEN'S STEPS TO
BREASTFEEDING SUCCESS

CHAPTER 1.
KNOW THAT BREASTMILK
IS NOT JUST FOOD

I'm going to start with a disclaimer: If you read this and think I
respect your decision, should you make it, to formula feed, you'
I have a reputation as a "breastfeeding supporter" like it's s............
aberrant. All pediatricians should be breastfeeding supporters, given
all the great benefits to our patients from breastmilk. So I ought to be
supporting it, and loudly. However, I will support whatever feeding method
you choose for your baby, as long as it's an informed decision. I want you
to start with the full story.

In return, I am willing to say something that struggling moms need to hear
more often: **Good mothering isn't just about breastfeeding.** And there is a
corollary to that. Breastfeeding isn't just about feeding our babies.

Does that make sense?

Let me explain by talking a bit about how we think about breastfeeding and
food and our babies. It's funny how more and more mothers are choosing
to breastfeed. But at the same time, it seems to me there's this part of
many of us that doesn't really believe our bodies—the same bodies that
created our beautiful children—can truly be capable of nourishing our
children properly. I hear it over and over and over again: *I'm not making
enough milk for him. Or my milk somehow isn't good enough for her—am I
eating the wrong foods? Feeding at the wrong times?* The worries are endless.
And I'll address all of these concerns. But first I want to back up for a
moment. Because at the heart of many of these worries is a turmoil that
has to do, really, with whether we believe we are "good-enough" mothers.
Are we doing this right? Are we doing enough? Too much? And during those
fragile days of new motherhood and breastfeeding, all of these worries
and hopes and contradictory feelings come crashing together in a way that
makes us doubt the most fundamental part of ourselves—our own bodies.

So let's back up and learn a bit about how our bodies and childbirth and
breastfeeding actually work from a physiological perspective. We worry
about whether our baby is feeding and growing as he "should." But too
often, we're not even quite sure what a "normal" baby is supposed to do.

What Is A Normal Newborn Baby Supposed To Do, Anyway?

Let's start there, at the moment when our babies are first born, so we can
examine this instinct to nurse and what it means.

In other words, what is a normal, full-term human infant supposed to do?

First of all, a human baby is supposed to be born vaginally. Yes, I know
that doesn't always happen, but we're just going to talk ideal for now. We
are supposed to be born vaginally because we need good bacteria. Human

babies are sterile, without bacteria, at birth. (I'll come back to this later in this book.) It's no accident that we are born near the anus, an area that has lots of bacteria, most of which are good and necessary for normal gut health and development of the immune system. And the bacteria that are there are mom's bacteria, bacteria she can provide antibodies against if the bacteria there aren't nice.

So in our ideal world, the baby is born vaginally. Then once baby is born, he is supposed to go directly to mom, right to her chest. The chest, right in between the breasts, is the natural habitat of the newborn baby. (It's interesting, I think, to note that our cardiac output, or how much blood we circulate in a given minute, is distributed to places that are important. Therefore, lots of blood goes to the kidney every minute, like 10 percent or so. And 20 percent goes to our brains. In a new mom, 23 percent of her blood goes to her chest—even more than goes to her brain. Clearly, after giving birth, the body thinks that place is really important. (And we should listen.)

That area of the chest gives heat. The baby can use mom to get warm. Babies have been using moms' bodies for temperature regulation for ages. Why would they stop? With all that blood flow, it's going to be warm. And so now, our "normal" newborn is on top of mom, snuggled. We have a brand new baby "on the warmer."

And do you know what? That child is not hungry. Honestly. Bringing a hungry baby into the world is a bad plan. (And really, if children were born hungry, can you please explain to me why my kids sucked the life force out of me in those last few weeks of pregnancy? They better have been getting food, or well, that would have been annoying and painful for nothing.)

Let me explain it like this: Every species has instinctual behaviors that allow the little ones to grow up to be big ones and keep the species going. Human babies are born into the world needing protection. Not food, at least not immediately. Human babies are not born hungry. But they are born needing protection from disease and from predators. Yes, predators. Our babies don't know they've been born into loving families in the 21st century—for all they know, it's the second century, and they are in a cave surrounded by tigers. And so our instinctive behaviors as baby humans need to help us stay protected. Luckily, babies get both disease protection *and* tiger protection from being on mom's chest. See why it's such a great place? Presumably, we gave babies some good bacteria when they arrived through the birth canal. That's the first step in disease protection. The next step is getting colostrum.

So a normal newborn baby snuggled on mom's chest will pick her head up, lick her hands, maybe nuzzle mom, lick her hands, and start to slide towards the breast. Yes, if left alone and to her natural instincts, the baby will perform this newborn crawl, or creep, toward mom's chest. And infants actually have a preference for contrasts between light and dark, and for circles over other shapes. Think about that...there's a dark circle not too far away.

Mom's sweat smells like amniotic fluid, and that smell is on the child's hands (because there's been no bath yet!). The baby uses that taste on her hands to follow mom's smell. Again, we're talking ideal here. The secretions coming from the glands on the areola (that dark circle) smell familiar, too, and help baby get to the breast to get the colostrum which is going to feed the good bacteria and keep baby protected from infection. The baby can attach by himself and get the colostrum he needs.

If you just need colostrum to feed bacteria (for disease protection) and not yourself, well, there doesn't have to be much. And there isn't. Because newborns aren't hungry. And because breastmilk is not just food.

Colostrum activates things in the baby's gut that make the thymus grow. The thymus is part of the immune system. Growing your thymus is important. Breastmilk equals big thymus, good immune system. Colostrum also has something called Secretory Immunoglobulin A (SIgA). SIgA is made in the first few days of life and is infection protection specifically from mom. Cells in mom's gut watch what's coming through, and if there's an infectious cell, a special cell in mom's gut called a plasma cell heads to the breast and helps the breast make SIgA in the milk to protect the baby. If mom and baby are together, like on mom's chest, then the baby is protected from what the two of them may be exposed to. Babies should be with mom.

Breastfeeding is normal. It's what babies are hardwired to do, in every sense of the word. Whether it's 2009 or 209, newborns would all do the same thing—try to find the breast. I don't know how much more clearly I can say this: Breastmilk isn't special sauce, a leg up, or a magic potion. It's not "best." It's normal. Just normal. Designed for the needs of a vulnerable human infant. And nothing else designed to replace it is normal.

What about the tigers? Define "tiger" however you want. But if you are a baby with no skills in self-protection, then staying with mom, having a grasp reflex, and having a startle reflex that helps you grab onto your mom all make sense.

Here's the other thing: Babies know the difference between a bassinette and a human chest. When newborn infants are separated from their mothers, they have a "despair-withdrawal" response. The despair part comes when they are alone, separated. The babies are vocally expressing their desire not to be tiger food. When they are picked up, they stop crying. They are protected, warm, and safe. Normal newborn babies want to be held.

So normal babies breastfeed, stay at the breast, and want to be held. That chest-to-chest contact is also helping brain development. As you are snuggling, your child is hooking up happy brain cells, and, hopefully, getting rid of the "eeeek" brain cells that tell her to cry. Breastfeeding, skin-to-skin, is brain-wiring. It's protection. Not just food.

Why go on and on about this? Because of what I said in the beginning— many mothers don't believe the body that created that beautiful baby is exclusively capable of feeding that same child. And so we are supplementing more and more with infant formulas—formulas designed to be food—even though our babies aren't just looking for food.

Why don't we trust our bodies postpartum? I don't know. But every day I hear a new mom needs to supplement with formula because "I am just not satisfying him."

To that, I almost always respond, "Of course you are." Newborn babies don't need to "eat" all the time—they need to be with you, at your chest, satisfying this instinct to seek protection.

A newborn baby at the breast is getting her immune system developed, activating her thymus, staying warm, feeling safe from predators, and wiring her brain. And (oh by the way) getting some food in the process. She is not "hungry"—she is obeying instinct, the instinct that allows us to survive and make more of us.

So your first step to achieve breastfeeding success: Understand that breastmilk is not just food. And your newborn is not hungry. Offer her the protection she needs, the chest-to-chest comfort she craves. And believe in the power of your own body.

Chapter 2.
Know Where You're Going
And Why

I'm going to switch gears for just a moment to explain that I am a runner, and have been since I was really little. Some families go on picnics, some go fishing...we went running. All the time. I am not good. I am not fast. But it's something I enjoy, and it doesn't require anything but a pair of shoes and the ability to put one foot in front of the other.

As an "experienced" runner, I have lately found myself with friends—in this case through social media, people across the world who I would totally hang out with if we were anywhere close to each other—who have just started running. And the (admittedly unsolicited) advice I found myself tweeting suddenly sounded to me a lot like the things I say to breastfeeding mothers. So to explain this step about the importance of knowing where you're going and why, I'd liked to share some of my exercise-inspired comparisons to breastfeeding.

Don't Make Decisions When You're Heading Uphill Into The Wind

- The first couple of weeks are hard, sometimes harder than you expect. That doesn't mean it isn't worth it.

- Celebrate the journey. Every day, every step is something to embrace and celebrate.

- Set reasonable expectations and embrace the experience day by day. (Yes, set long-term goals, but don't let those be the only milestones you congratulate yourself for achieving.)

- Your friends probably will have different experiences than you. Some may be faster. Some may cover more ground. That's okay. You aren't doing this for them.

- Pain means something is wrong. Yes, you read that correctly, and it's important, so I'll say it again. *Pain means something is wrong.* You can expect it to be hard, you might be sore, and maybe you might feel tender. But pain is not cool. It means something is wrong. You need to listen and find what needs to be fixed. (More on this from the breastfeeding end in another chapter!)

- Embarking on any new adventure that requires time and energy also requires support. Find somebody to share the experience with you, so they can be a cheerleader and give you that push when you need it. And then pay it forward.

- You don't need fancy equipment. You need your body and a good attitude. (Admittedly, I do have lots of fancy equipment that I don't need. I'm fine with that, too.)

- Don't make important decisions while going uphill into the wind. Remember this: When it's easiest to stop, when you're tired and it's hard, and you can't go one more minute into that headwind, wait until you turn the corner and catch your breath before deciding what you can and cannot accomplish.

- Attitude is everything here. If you think it's going to be awful and overwhelming and impossible, it will. If you go into it knowing that you are strong and having confidence in your body, it will go so much better.

- Find your mantra. My favorite is *"I am deceptively strong,"* and I'd like to say this is the one that pulls me through the hard times. Unfortunately, the truth is the one that has stuck with me more is the advice given to me at the nine–mile mark of a 15–mile race I was doing with my dad. As I was complaining that we were going too fast, he said, *"Shut up and run."* Yes, I guess I do come back to that one most often. Sometimes you need to just shut up and run. (My mother, however, has a nicer approach. *"I figure it's been a good day if I just cover the ground,"* she says. I like that one, too.)

To get back to the point, why all this talk about running? Because when you're running, you begin at the beginning. Yes, you have a goal in mind. But truly, you take it one step at a time. And at the end, hopefully, you celebrate every step you made. And that is what I want for you on your breastfeeding journey.

So let us begin at the beginning. Why breastfeed? Or to put it another way, know *why* you're doing this. To that end, here are my top five reasons why breastmilk will always be better than formula!

Why Breastmilk Will Always Be Better Than Formula

1. Protection Against Infection

Children who are formula-fed are at significant risk for infection. We have just come to accept that infants get RSV, rotavirus, and ear infections. They are not supposed to be diseases of infants, but in the U.S.A., the largest consumer of formulas worldwide, we hospitalize many, many, many infants each winter with those diseases. The great majority of those infants are formula-fed. In fact, the number one risk factor for kids getting ear infections is bottle feeding—not day care, not smoke exposure, but formulas. Think about the loss of work, the exposure to antibiotics, the midnight purchases of medicine for fever and rehydration solutions, and the visits to me that could be avoided if more families chose to breastfeed their infants.

You see, infection-fighting cells of the body are present in abundance in breastmilk and are not found at all in formula. So children who are formula-fed are not just at risk for ear infections, but also for diarrhea (from rotavirus, *E. coli,* cholera, Giardia) and respiratory infections (like RSV, influenza, H. flu, pneumococcus). Plus, formula-fed kids get more meningitis (from H. flu, pneumococcus, herpes, and group B strep).

2. Protection Against Inflammation

Breastmilk contains a myriad of factors that allow the body to fight infection and other invaders without inflammation. And inflammation in the infant gut is really undesirable at any point, but especially for the premature infant. Factors in breastmilk protect premature infants from a potentially fatal gut complication called necrotizing enterocolitis (NEC). Children born at 30 weeks of gestation have a six–to ten–fold increase in their risk for NEC if they are formula-fed.

3. Protection Against Cancer—For Mom!

We definitely do not talk about this enough. Breastfeeding is beneficial for mothers. A study done in 2002 found that for every 12 months a mom breastfeeds, her risk of breast cancer decreases 4.3 percent as compared to women who never nursed. Another study found a 54 percent reduction for women who breastfed for greater than 24 months. In a time when we see pink ribbons everywhere, this important protection from breastfeeding should NOT be discounted or downplayed. Breastfeeding is breast cancer prevention!

4. Protection Over the Lifespan

The American Academy of Pediatrics Task Force on Sudden Infant Death Syndrome (SIDS) affirmed in 2011 what research has told us for some time: Breastfed children are less likely to die of SIDS. An important aspect of their recommendation for protection against SIDS was the strong endorsement of breastfeeding.

Also crucial for lifetime health is the role breastfeeding plays in obesity prevention. Breastfed kids have less obesity as they enter kindergarten. This is so important that everyone from the U.S. Centers for Disease Control and Prevention (CDC) to the White House to the U.S. Surgeon General are all talking about it.

5. A Consistent Recipe

Breastmilk has had the same recipe for many, many, many years. It hasn't needed a fanfare of advertising for every new ingredient because the ingredients haven't needed to change. The celebrating that formula companies do about the improvements in their product are really what happens when a deficit is fixed. Formula companies realized that their product needed to be fortified with vitamin D when kids started having seizures from low calcium levels. They tried to help combat adult high blood pressure problems with a type of formula low in sodium until kids started having seizures from low sodium levels. When there wasn't enough iron in their product, they found out after many kids became anemic, and iron-deficiency anemia, as we have learned, has had developmental consequences. Plus, formulas in powder form have the potential to be contaminated with bacteria. (The ready-to-feed and concentrate are sterilized, but powders aren't. The great majority of formula recalls have been because powdered forms were contaminated with potentially harmful bacteria.) Other ingredients, found in breastmilk, are still missing. In the future, we may see other additions to formula like infection-fighting oligosaccharides, insulin, and prebiotics. That means they are not in the recipe now.

So What if All the Ingredients in Breastmilk Got in Formula Some Day...

So let's say they get all the ingredients in breastmilk (all the white blood cells, antibodies, anti-inflammatory cells, and biologically active compounds that are so important to our children's health) in formula... would breastmilk still be better?

Yes. Of course. The milk a mom makes for her baby is perfect for her child. Nobody else can ever make a more perfect food. The antibodies in a mom's milk are specific to the viruses and bacteria that mom and baby came into contact with during that day. The composition of the milk varies from the beginning of the day to the end of the day and from the beginning of the feeding to its end. It changes to meet a growing baby's needs and is flavored with foods that mom ate, making every mouthful of food different and perfect for that baby. No formula company can ever make a more perfect food for your baby than you can as the baby's mother.

(And for those of you who find you are medically unable to breastfeed—and to all of you who may someday know someone who is medically unable to breastfeed—I want to say again that it isn't just breastmilk that makes a child special. If you try to nurse and are unable to, or if you have a medical problem that makes nursing impossible, then take heart in the fact that formulas now have the nutrition children need and that you tried to breastfeed. Your children are better for the effort. And they can still have the important skin-to-skin contact, no matter how you are feeding! Keep up that effort!)

Step number two to achieving breastfeeding success: **Know where you are going and why. You are breastfeeding your baby because it is the most natural, perfectly designed food for your human infant and because your body was designed to keep the connection you developed during pregnancy and make a wonderful transition after birth. Yes, have a goal. But always remember why you're doing this to begin with, and celebrate EVERY step along the way.**

CHAPTER 3.
TAKE THE FIRST STEP.
AND THEN BABY STEPS.

So, about that first step? When it comes to breastfeeding (and maybe running, too, for that matter), some people think it encompasses everything from learning the best technique to buying the fancy equipment. I, on the other hand, am a pretty literal person, so I'm going to define the "first step" as the moment your newborn baby reaches your nipple. (Everything that comes before, I'll call preparation.) So...you've read everything you could about breastfeeding; you've perhaps taken a class and received gifts to help your breastfeeding progress. But really, it's all about this moment, when your baby has finally arrived and is snuggled to your chest.

Yes, there are some things you can and should do at this very moment and in the days that immediately follow to ensure your breastfeeding success. But before I describe them, let me say that if you're already past this point—if you're struggling with a six-day-old baby who was born by C-section and didn't see you or your breast for hours afterward; if your three-week-old was supplemented in the hospital nursery on day two; if your five-week-old already loves her pacifier and you wonder if that's why she's been so demanding at the breast...whatever...please know that none of the information that immediately follows is meant to "make" you feel guilty or imply that you did something "wrong."

(And may I digress slightly here? Your emotions are yours. Nobody but you can own or change them. I have very much wanted to "make" people feel things—a guy in the seventh grade who I really liked; my husband who totally messed up my birthday; and oh, there are many others. You know what, though? You can't do it. You can't "make" people feel anything—happy, guilty, miserable, remorseful, anything. And no one can "make" you feel these things, either. Own your emotions. Don't give them away.)

And just to make my view perfectly clear here, I'll offer another disclaimer, or perhaps an admission: Many "breastfeeding failures" fall directly at the hands of healthcare providers, hospitals, and other people who should know better. You can read "Temple of Doom" later in this book to get my take on that. But for now, I'll just make it clear I know quite well the factors that contribute to breastfeeding failure are far too often outside of the mother's control. And finally, I do know some women just can't breastfeed. If donor milk isn't available, we need to have substitutes that support the growth of our children. I'm not saying formula is evil or judging the moms that use it. I, for one, am grateful it exists.

So, now back to our regular programming...if you are struggling to breastfeed and you're already past the first hours and days of your baby's life, please know we'll get to you in just a moment, and you can get back on track. But for now, let's imagine the freshly newborn baby. That freshly newborn baby, remember from Chapter One, goes directly to mom's chest.

In an Ideal World, How Does the Perfect Breastfeeding Relationship Begin?

In this perfect world I'm describing next, you would have a vaginal delivery without an epidural and be given your precious little one right as they were delivered. He or she would be placed right on your chest, immediately. The baby could be dried, assigned APGAR scores (a score that tells us how the baby is transitioning to their new world), and have their initial assessment done right there on your chest, while skin-to-skin in the best place for that baby in the entire world.

Then, your little one would obey instinct, head raised and hand in mouth, and kicking gently would move towards the breast. The scent on the baby's hands would serve as a road map to the areola, and free from any mittens or covers, they would grab to help pull out the nipple. The baby's chin would touch your breast. The baby would latch without causing pain and get several swallows of colostrum. All this would happen in the first hour. The birth weight, length, footprints, and whatever else we medical professionals feel needs to be done are done after the first feeding. The staff would all be supportive and would know what a good latch looks like. (For more on this, see the next chapter, which goes into more specific detail about latches and nipple pain.)

It could happen. Of course, I do know the ideal doesn't always happen. But it's nice to know what it looks like, don't you think?

Sleep—Part 1: I'm So Tired; Why Won't My Baby Stop Crying?

As a pediatrician, an advocate for my youngest and most vulnerable patients, I would be remiss in a chapter about taking these first steps, about surviving those first long and often overwhelming days of nursing a newborn baby, if I did not address an important aspect of your own health as a new mom—sleep deprivation. The simple fact is that sleep deprivation is one of the hardest parts of being a new parent, and I certainly will come back to this theme of baby's sleep habits and the question of "crying it out," several more times throughout this book. It's an important topic. And so I'll start sharing my view on infant sleep right now, as we take these first steps, because this issue is so fundamental to achieving breastfeeding success. Remember: It's about taking one step at a time.

The question I get frequently from new parents goes something like this: *I'm so tired, why won't my baby stop crying?* And so I offer an approach to crying in the breastfed newborn. And, being me, I offer it by first asking a simple, biological question: Why do babies cry? (Or, as is often the question posed by a bleary-eyed, sleep-deprived parent: Why won't my baby stop crying?) Contrary to what you might expect, this is not an easy question.

For babies, crying can lead to a desired result, like having his needs met. Or it can lead to a truly undesired result, like being abused.

Human infants are the only infants in which crying can persist once the cause of the crying is fixed. For example, only human infants will cry while in the arms of a caregiver. And then that crying can continue independently of the original cause. It's this crying that gets us worried: *No matter what we do, he doesn't seem to stop.*

Some have theorized that this sort of infant crying is a way to relieve tension and excess energy associated with being a helpless and relatively immobile being. I remember hearing that somewhere in my education: *Let them cry, it's good for their lungs...sometimes they need to blow off steam."* You could see how it may be linked to how we feel as adults when we cry. But studies have been done to look at newborns raised in non-Western cultures, and those newborns are healthy and psychologically sound *without* crying, suggesting that babies don't need to cry to relieve tension.

Research (and practical experience) suggests that crying happens because of pain, hunger, and a need for attention. Crying and infant well-being are very much linked.

But the most important cause of crying in an otherwise healthy newborn appears to be being alone. Crying is a survival tactic when our kids are alone, yet we are encouraged as part of our culture to ignore this crying. When we ignore it, the crying can escalate and gets very hard to stop. Therefore, our parenting culture is an important contributor to crying in our infants. We carry our babies much less than our non-Western counterparts. In fact, in randomized controlled trials, even a little bit of extra holding has been shown to make a huge difference in the amount of crying a newborn will do. We also know from research that crying is likely lessened because the physiologic state that goes with being held increases opioid release and increases serotonin.

Crying is a means of communication from the newborn that says, *"I need something."* However, crying likely developed as a means of occasional communication. Vocalizing displeasure and need may get mom's attention, but it's also a good way to get the attention of predators. Using it as a consistent means of communication wouldn't make a lot of sense. Smell and vision were probably meant to be the main ways of communication, with vocalizations being last resort.

In our culture, instead of addressing crying early to prevent the newborn from being attacked by predators, we may actually just ignore it, or worse, go to extreme ways of getting it to stop. Ignoring crying (**unless you just need to walk away**) is not going to make anything better. In non-Western cultures, the response to crying is immediate and rates of infant crying are much lower.

So, my approach to a crying breastfed baby:

I used to work in an ICU, so for my first approach, even after all these years as a generalist, I still go to *"Is the baby sick or not sick?"* Then we look for indicators of infant well-being: Is the baby gaining weight? Is she maintaining a normal temperature, respiratory and heart rate? Is the child eating normally? Is she showing signs of illness, like lethargy? Does the crying have a pattern (as it would with colic) or is it consistent (which could mean pathology)? Is the baby consolable? Inconsolable babies should be evaluated. So should one who isn't gaining weight, is demonstrating signs of illness, isn't eating well...you get the point. Call your provider.

Things to think about if we're in the "not sick" category:

- The child is hungry. We have some need to schedule feedings in our culture, but we have the ready-made answer right at our breasts. If the baby is crying and the breast soothes that crying, well then, breastfeed! Schedules. Yuck.

- The baby loves you. You are not a failure because your child doesn't want to be separated from you. You are a rock star. Just because our culture says our babies should be able to be away from us doesn't make it true.

Things you can think about, but that probably aren't the cause of crying:

- I'm eating something that disagrees with the baby. I have to admit, I have a hard time with this one, scientifically speaking. Taste is developed long before delivery and breastmilk provides an array of flavors. Keep that in mind before we blame what you are eating. I'm not saying what you are eating isn't the cause, but it's not as likely as we seem to make it. What do you think mothers in Mexico, Greece, Thailand, or Italy eat while nursing? They certainly aren't staying away from spices or garlic. We think what you eat during lactation helps babies adapt to their native cuisine. There are people who know their children have a specific sensitivity to something—I'm not saying this can't be true. But it's over-blamed.

- Reflux? True gastroesophageal reflux disease is rare. Reflux is not a common cause of unexplained crying or distressed behavior in otherwise healthy infants. Reflux is a normal physiological process occurring several times per day in healthy infants, children, and adults. It's diagnosed a lot, but the research does not support it as a cause of crying.

What else it may be:

- Oversupply or the coughing, choking, unhappy breastfed child. (I write about this more in Part Two, where I examine breastfeeding issues and help provide answers.)

- Nicotine: In several studies the prevalence of unexplained crying was higher among infants of smoking mothers, but less among breastfed infants.

- Withdrawal: Remember the part about opioid and serotonin involvement in calming crying? Well, the opposite can be true. Babies withdrawing from opioids are cranky. And there are reports of "colic" symptoms in children of mothers who were on the drug class of SSRIs (Prozac, Zoloft, Paxil) during pregnancy.

- Cow's milk protein in the diet. That's a rare thing. Studies shows about 4 percent of children actually have a cow's milk protein allergy. But it is a recognized cause of crying.

- Colic: Believe it or not, this is defined as an infant "who, otherwise healthy and well-fed, has paroxysms of irritability, fussing, or crying lasting for a total of three hours a day and occurring on more than three days in any one week for a period of three weeks" (Wessel et al., 1954). In other words, this is what we call a "diagnosis of exclusion," meaning we've looked at everything else and can't find an answer. In other words, crying for no good reason. I have to be honest here. I don't like this diagnosis.

SO WHAT DO WE DO TO FIX IT?

Well, I have to say that when there is not a medical reason for the infant's distress, all answers point to holding the baby and being responsive to crying. Does that sound too simple? It's certainly not an easy answer when you consider how demanding and *needy* our newborn human infants can be. But it definitely does answer the needs of a crying newborn human infant...and in a way that truly understands and respects those primal needs. (Some parents answer this need, and keep their hands free, by baby-wearing. But if you don't want to baby-wear, just holding them more helps tremendously.)

Now here I have to add: If the crying is too much, if you truly cannot handle another moment without doing something rash and regrettable, please **walk away** and find someone to care for the baby until you are better. If you don't get better, please find help.

What I've Learned From You About Those First Days

Now that you've seen, hopefully, what the ideal first step in your breastfeeding relationship looks like, I'd like to take a quick peek at some of the things that interfere with it, things we'll deal with in more depth in other parts of the book.

Speaking with my patients and at conferences across the country, these are among the several themes that have clearly emerged about the barriers facing new breastfeeding moms:

- A misperception of what a normal newborn baby does in those first few days. (Hunger vs. instinct, which we've already discussed in Chapter One. Hopefully, you won't fall victim to that particular trap!)

- The complications that mode of delivery and delivery interventions can make.

- A general lack of support. From everybody.

- Words like "starving baby" and "dehydration," which are scary and effective in making people change their feeding plans.

- A line of demarcation between colostrum and milk "coming in." I think we need to explore this a little, and we will in Chapter 9.

- And the ever present "Three Bs"—blood sugar, birthweight, and bilirubin, which I'll explore more in depth in another geeky medical chapter.

The thing I find most frustrating about all of these chapters is a sense that, as new mothers, we so often feel a lack of control over what happens to our bodies and our babies—what happens, how it happens, and what our part is in it. Informed consent is a basic principle of medicine and ethics, and it's discouraging to me that so many actions and interventions when it comes to newborn care seem to be done without informed consent.

With that said, I'll add that what makes me just feel happy all over is the fact that most new mothers DO overcome these "first steps" issues and go on to successfully breastfeed for however long they chose. So take heart! Learn everything you can.

And remember our third step to breastfeeding success: **Take the first step. Skin-to-skin, follow your baby's lead. And then take baby steps, remembering to celebrate each and every one of them!**

CHAPTER 4.
TRUST YOUR BABY,
TRUST YOURSELF

Sound simple enough? Well, in the early days of establishing your breastfeeding relationship, I have to tell you that this whole trust thing is harder than it sounds. I mean, before you got started, you might have thought something like this: Your body makes human milk, your baby drinks human milk—how hard can it be, right? But guess what? This whole breastfeeding thing indeed can be harder than it looks, and all too often is even harder than it should be.

Really, this step involves trusting several things on several levels. The first is trusting your body to actually make the milk your baby needs. *My milk hasn't come in yet,* I often hear from panicked moms, frequently when their babies are only hours old, already ready to supplement with "just one bottle" that I'll warn about more in the next chapter. For now, I'll remind you: Your baby was not born into this world in need of food, but instead in need of protection. And the colostrum your body produces is enough for those first postpartum days.

So that's the first part—to take a breath and trust the process. Your body and your baby **will** give clear signals if all is not going as it should, and I will outline for you exactly how to read and understand those signals later in the chapter. But trust your body.

The second step, trusting your baby, is two-fold. By this, I do mean to trust your baby to find your source of nourishment and establish a proper latch (which, again, we'll talk about in more detail). But the second part is to also trust your baby's signals when it comes to feeding—as you'll see, the baby drives the bus here. You need to trust that your baby is not being manipulative, demanding, or unreasonable when she cries and nurses frequently. Really. Breastfeeding is very much a supply-and-demand relationship, and when your baby needs to nurse more frequently, it means you need to trust her enough to understand that it's because she's urging your body to up its milk production to meet her needs.

So the trust involves a lot of layers.

How New Moms End Up Confused, Rather Than Confident

Let's start with you, and the trust you need to establish to move forward. All too frequently I see mothers three–to five–days postpartum who are simply dazed and confused. Their hospital stay has been difficult. Whenever their baby cries, everyone gives different advice. They are tired. They are worn down. They are unsure. They have lost their confidence. They are focused not on their bodies, not on their babies, but simply on the *numbers*. What numbers? Oh, trust me, there are a lot of numbers involved when you have a newborn baby. Numbers measuring everything: bilirubin, weight loss, stool diapers, wet diapers, minutes at the breast (minutes at the left breast, and minutes at the right breast), hours between feedings, time of last feeding, time to next feeding, hours slept, and hours not slept.

Add to that a dazzling array of instruction for this helpless new person: cord care, diaper care, skin care, and bathing, and the often scary warnings about sleep placement. Don't forget postpartum care for mom, conflicting (and often unsolicited) opinions from doctors, nurses, lactation consultants, family members, and friends...and you have a recipe for "dazed and confused."

I have to tell you that it's heartbreaking watching a new mother in my exam room, tearful, trying to wade through what she wants to say and ask. Words like *powerless, scared, anguish,* and *failure* run through the subtext of these conversations. All of that information, all of that advice, all of those warnings—even if given with the best intentions—has created a truly and deeply hard situation.

It's really no wonder that the first large drop-off in breastfeeding rates happens in the first week.

So, what can we do?

Well, I love to say *"Worry in order."* In other words, prioritize your fears. What do you need to worry about *right* now? It's a simple philosophy, really, to help decide what needs to come next. For example, it does us no good to worry about college when our beautiful new baby still hasn't learned the fine art of potty training. It does us no good to worry about potty training when the umbilical cord hasn't even fallen off. You get the picture—it's too easy to live your life all in the one moment (and even in the one crummy, difficult moment). We don't need that, honestly—and especially in the days immediately after giving birth.

So, here is my advice to those dazed and confused new moms in those foggy postpartum days: Look at your baby. That's right, look at your baby. Soak in the newborn smell, admire the incredible delicacy of her hands. Watch the fun tongue movements and facial expressions. Enjoy watching that special peace on the face of a baby who is sleeping. Celebrate that *you* are the one who brought that beautiful baby into the world. And then breathe. Just breathe.

All those numbers, all that confusion. Let it go. What numbers are important? If it were up to me, all the clocks in the homes of new parents would be turned off. Rules about how long to feed aren't helpful. The number of feedings is important, but counting them doesn't take a clock. And the hormone that allows milk to be released from the breast, oxytocin, is exquisitely sensitive to stress. Makes perfect sense, too. If you could release milk in front of a predator (You know my preference is a tiger. Why? It works—easy to picture, hard to forget.) in a place that really wasn't safe, the creatures trying to get you could use a trail of milk to track you down. Less stress, more oxytocin, more milk release, and happier mom and baby.

What other tigers can we tackle as we worry in order? Well, visitors come to mind. I get it—everyone wants to meet the new baby. We take such good care of you when you're pregnant, throwing showers, opening doors, giving up our seats, or whatever, so you can be comfortable. Then you have the baby and things change. I feel especially sorry for those mothers who have C-sections. Really, I think we'd pay more attention to you if you had your appendix out. Mothers who have a C-section had *surgery*, no way around that. After we have surgery, we relax and recover. But now you have to care for a new baby.

No matter how your baby was born, you still have to recover and come to understand and embrace your birth experience, even if it was absolutely perfect, but especially if it wasn't what you planned. If you have visitors on top of that, hopefully, they are willing to help. If they aren't, or if they expect you to entertain, have a clean house, or even have clean clothes on, maybe they should wait until you and your new family are recovered and ready to have people come over. I love dad to step in here. He can protect his new family and decide when visitors are welcome.

Now, about that baby? How can you trust a baby to eat when she needs to eat, especially when it seems like she wants to sleep all the time?

Waking a sleeping baby is no fun. A baby who hasn't demonstrated feeding cues and is woken up anyway to eat might just snuggle against the breast and sleep. The breast is warm, smells good and familiar, represents safety and comfort, and is a neat place to fall back asleep. Babies should be fed on cue. (Trust, remember?) It's easier on everyone if the baby is feeding when there is an interest is feeding.

Signals Your Baby Is Getting Enough Milk

The most important signal that your baby is drinking and digesting milk is that she is pooping. The first poop from a breastfed baby is black and tarry from the colostrum. Then it becomes green and tarry and less sticky, then brown, then yellow.

Other important signals: You feel your milk let down when your baby feeds (although this may not happen with every mother). You can hear or see your baby swallowing. Your baby seems content after feeding.

Ask for help if your baby does not seem to be getting milk. Particularly, if your baby is not producing poop, ask for help.

Now, there are cases where babies sleep and sleep and sleep, and make everybody nervous. The best indicator that a baby is transferring enough milk is stool output. The first milk, colostrum, is full of sugars called oligosaccharides. They are a form of insoluble fiber, meaning they aren't digested, and, therefore, they act as a great laxative. The more colostrum a baby transfers, the more stool is produced. That stool goes from black and tarry stuff I swear you could build houses with, to green and tarry and less sticky, to brown, to yellow. And we love yellow stool on day four, maybe day five of life. I feel as if I can turn perfectly intelligent people into "poop watchers." As long as your very sleepy baby is stooling and moving the meconium out, then milk is transferring and all is well. **No stool output and you should ask for help.** Seriously, ask. There are armies of people out there who want to help. I know I have to give most new moms permission to get that help, so I am. **Ask for help.** In fact, in most prenatal breastfeeding classes I teach, I have moms raise their hands and promise me they will ask for help. Those of us trained and passionate about helping breastfeeding mothers want to hear from you. We are the hired help.

Why harp on this? Because another reason I see "dazed and confused" mothers in the immediate newborn period is that they are under the impression that pain is a part of breastfeeding. Not true. I can't tell you how many arguments I've had with new (and experienced) mothers where they think pain in the first few days of nursing is to be expected. Or that pain with the initial few sucks of the latch is normal. Now tell me: When is pain normal? It's a terrifically designed part of the human body, which acts as a signal that something is wrong.

Pain is not normal. Pressure, soreness, maybe. But pain? No way. Remember: This is about trusting your body. If your body is in pain,

listen. Something is wrong, and I'll tell you, it's probabl\
Because here's the thing—nobody can look at the latch\
looks fine." Whether the latch is "fine" depends on your\
baby latches. **If the latch hurts, no matter what it lo\
outside, something is wrong.**

Too often we see the nipple and surrounding areola as a bull's-eye. And we treat it as such, trying to aim the baby's mouth to be centered over the nipple. What really needs to happen is that the baby's tongue needs to compress the milk ducts, which are behind the areola and nipple, and compress them from below the nipple, not from the center of the bull's-eye target. When we center the baby's mouth with the nipple right in the middle, the baby will scrape the nipple for a few sucks before the tongue gets into the right spot. That hurts and **pain is a sign that something is wrong.**

If the latch keeps hurting, it's a lose-lose situation. The baby is not transferring milk because the tongue is in the wrong place, and you are getting beat up, experiencing pain and nipple trauma. The baby is hungry, you're in pain—who wins? Nobody. The latch is not supposed to hurt. If it does, please, please, please ask for help. Pain is a tiger. It inhibits oxytocin and impairs milk release. Getting the picture? Ask for help if something hurts.

See what I mean? Trust your body. When your body is sending you pain signals, listen. Ask for help.

And if everything is going well, well, you need to trust that, too. Yes, trust. Just breathe in that newborn baby smell and trust.

How the Breast Makes Milk

Okay, so how the heck are you going to trust your body to make milk for that beautiful baby if you don't even know how the whole process works? Of course, you could just believe me and trust! But I thought it might be even more fun to walk you through the process, to talk a bit about how a woman's body actually produces milk, the perfect food for her baby. And hopefully, it will help you understand why it's so important not **just** to trust your body, but also to trust your baby.

The breast is an interesting organ (yes, it is!) in that much of the development happens during a particular phase of life—pregnancy. During pregnancy, the breast grows by making more ducts and enhancing its supporting structures ("stroma"). These structures that need to be set up for the production of milk are complete around 16 weeks of pregnancy.

your breasts are ready to make milk at 16 weeks of pregnancy, y don't we see the milk being secreted? Some women do, but for the vast majority of us, the milk is not secreted because of high levels of the hormones progesterone and estrogen, and a hormone from the placenta called "human placental lactogen." In addition, progesterone sensitizes the milk-producing cells of the breast to the effects of insulin, a crucial hormone in the production of milk. And thyroid hormone (who thought the thyroid would make a difference in breastfeeding?) increases breast sensitivity to the effects of prolactin, the most essential hormone in making breastmilk.

At birth, everything changes. That's because the source of progesterone, estrogen, and human placental lactogen is the placenta, and we aren't going to have it around much longer. The removal of the placenta allows milk secretion to begin. The hormones that held milk secretion in check are gone. The production of milk at this stage is dependant on the appropriate development of the ducts, stroma, and the interplay of the important hormones that create milk.

Milk production at birth and for a few days afterwards is dependent on hormones, not on milk removal or a good latch or anything else we are used to talking about when we talk about having a good milk supply. It is extremely unusual for mothers to have "no milk" in these first few days if everything else has been going along fine. Since the milk production is small in the first few days, and the breasts aren't as full as they will be at postpartum day four to six, it may be pretty easy to convince yourself you have no milk and start second guessing your ability to feed your baby. It may even be enough for you to believe that your baby needs to be supplemented with something other than your own milk.

Since colostrum, the first recipe of milk that you make, is a great laxative, you know you are making enough milk when the baby starts to stool.

A few days after birth, the endocrine process of making milk (the removal of some hormones and the increase in others) gives way to an "autocrine" process, where the more milk that is removed is a signal for more milk to be made. This is the part that is dependent on the latch—good technique resulting in good milk transfer from the breast to the baby.

Prolactin is the hormone responsible for making milk. It is released only when the baby suckles effectively at the breast. Prolactin is an interesting hormone (if you find hormones interesting) in that it is the only one to be constantly inhibited. Other hormones are regulated, so if they get too high, regulating hormones come and keep them from being produced. Conversely, if they get too low, other regulating hormones help more of them to be created. Prolactin, though, is constantly held in check by dopamine. Suckling starts, dopamine levels decrease, and prolactin surges out of the brain, only to be inhibited again by dopamine. This prolactin surging happens during the whole time the baby is feeding. The normal pattern for prolactin release while breastfeeding is the pulsing, surging secretion multiple times during a feeding.

The other really important hormone, oxytocin, can be released from your brain under a variety of situations, including orgasm, birth, and suckling at the breast. Oxytocin is responsible for the milk ejection reflex or "let-down" that allows milk to be released from the breast. (I'm not much of a fan of the term "let-down." I very much prefer the term milk ejection reflex. Seriously, who needs another let down?) Oxytocin is inhibited by stress. Bummer, since stress seems to be everywhere sometimes.

Breastmilk production is regulated the way we'd expect. Too much milk sitting in the breast causes the release of the "feedback inhibitor of lactation," which tells your body to stop making more milk, so your breasts don't explode. You make more milk by removing more milk. The milk removal keeps the feedback inhibitor of lactation (FIL) away, so you continually make the milk your baby needs. Frequent milk removal helps create a robust milk supply.

The feedback inhibitor of lactation makes appropriate management of engorgement so very important. If you are engorged, your body will sense that your breasts are too full and slow production of more milk. Getting milk removed during those days where you are really full helps establish your milk supply and keeps your body from releasing the FIL hormone, which may hurt your supply. Early, unrestricted feedings are the key to establishing a good milk supply. Getting off to this good start is so important.

SLEEP—PART 2: SLEEP DEPRIVATION AND THE TEMPTATION TO "CRY IT OUT"

Before closing out this section on knowing the roadblocks, I need to come back, yet again, to this important issue of sleep habits—and how you, as a new parent, can also trust your baby and trust your own instincts when it comes to this topic. Why is this so important? I've said it before and I'll say it again: Sleep deprivation is one of the hardest parts of being a new parent. Or an experienced one. Or being a person in general.

And the truth is, I would guess that most parents who are trying a "crying it out" method are doing so because it's what they believe they are "supposed" to do...even if not responding to their baby's cry is going against every instinct they have as a parent. Why? My guess is it's because they are tired and other things they have tried haven't worked.

To get to the heart of the matter, I think we are placing 21st century values onto an infant who is obeying instinct. Maybe we don't understand that instinct. But we have to understand the way we do things—the way we understand the world—is a new idea, and our babies are born without knowing our new ideas. It's a new idea, biologically speaking, to believe that babies are perfectly safe from predators and are simply crying to manipulate us. But guess what? The babies we bring into this world don't know about the way we do things, what we believe. They are programmed to do things that normal, vulnerable human babies have been doing for all time.

Let me explain it like this: Human babies are really vulnerable. If you've ever seen what baby elephants or horses can do at birth, you know they can walk shortly after birth and are running soon afterwards. Why can't humans do that? Well, if we waited until the brain was mature enough for our kids to walk, never mind run, the baby's head would be too big to come out safely. We don't need to run to stay safe. Our gestation period is designed to make sure that our kids arrive in the world with their future intact—our kids arrive in the world when it's safest for the brain to come out.

Our children arrive in the world as the most neurologically immature primate of them all, and remain the most dependent on a caregiver for the longest period of time. Our kids can't keep themselves warm, get food, walk, speak, or reason. They can't manipulate us, and they can't consciously choose to make you look like a bad parent.

What do we know about their sleep patterns? Well, they need to be near a caregiver—mostly mom. It makes sense if you think about it. This immature baby, with little in the way of self-preservation skills, needs to hang out with the source of food and warmth, with the person who is most likely to wake up to meet the needs they express in the middle of the night. There are beautiful videos of moms and babies who are almost totally in sync in terms of sleep cycles, showing them waking at about the same time several times during the night, with mom responding to the baby, and the baby, who rarely cries, getting their multiple needs met.

Normal babies sleep during the day and are up at night. This is normal and expected, and there is nothing we can do to change that. The predators that hunt humans hunt at night. Instinctively, that means they should be up at night and sleep when the threat is less. That also means that parents need to sleep when the baby is sleeping to avoid all the great things that go along with sleep deprivation.

The littlest kids are not crying for any other reason than to communicate displeasure with something. And it gets our attention. So much so, that

I think kids develop a parent-specific pitch that affects us more than any other person listening to that same cry. Smart plan—it keeps the kids safe and lets them know that their parents are there and meeting their needs.

Sleep training techniques that suggest you allow children to cry to learn to soothe themselves have never been shown to do anything good for children. They may get the kids to sleep, and, therefore, help the parents sleep, but they have been associated with attachment issues, behavior problems, and anxiety. There is no emotional, social, or intellectual benefit to the kids, nor has it ever been shown to help us develop into healthy adult sleepers.

There is a phenomenon called "learned helplessness" that comes from some experiments that found that if you ask enough and never get what you need, you stop asking. You learn, in the case of a crying baby, not that you are "soothed," but that nobody is coming. That's not something, I imagine, most people want their kids to learn, no matter how tired you are. And ask yourself—can you soothe yourself? I'm 40 something and I'm pretty sure I can't go without shoe shopping or an episode of *True Blood*. I see commercial after commercial for Ambien and Lunesta, so I'm pretty sure the adult population has sleep problems. Plus, as an adult, we can get up, read, watch TV, get on Facebook, get warm milk, or call a friend. People who don't feel safe in their environment, like those suffering from depression, will often say they can't sleep or can't stay asleep.

What can our kids do if they can't sleep, if they don't feel safe in their environment? They can't take medication, read, watch TV, or do anything like we can. My advice, if the kids are crying, is to go in and comfort them. Nurse them if you are nursing. Snuggle and enjoy.

I hear all the time "OOOOH don't do that, once you give in, it'll never stop." Sure it will. In fact, there are going to be days when your children are going to be embarrassed to be seen in public with you. Their childhood will be over before you know it. Enjoy your time with them while it lasts.

So step four to a successful breastfeeding relationship: Trust your body. Trust your baby. Know and understand the signals that are given when everything is going right, and when things might be going wrong. Be ready to ask for help. But trust that you and your baby **CAN** do this.

WISDOM OF ON-DEMAND FEEDING...FROM A POET. AN OLD ONE.

P.S. We didn't start scheduling our kids until the 19th century, and then learned that maybe we were wrong about that in early 20th century. Maybe we should have listened to this guy:

And I, for suckling, no fix'd hour prescribe;

This Nature teaches best the nursing tribe:

Let her your mistress be; and when, with cries

The hungry child demand his due supplies,

Forbear not you the wish'd relief to bring

But, for his use, unlock the sacred spring:

Nor then be loath your snowy breast to bare,

That he may suck, and streaming fragrance share.

Sainte-Marthe, Paedotrophia, 1584

Chapter 5.
Be Prepared For
The Roadblocks

It's time for me to go back to the running analogy I started a few chapters back. I have to admit even if you're just putting one foot in front of the other, no experienced runner heads out without some sort of idea of what to expect on the run. Perhaps it's planning the route; maybe it's just checking the weather report. But it's always good to know what sort of roadblocks might await you.

In this case, this is going to be a bit of a long chapter. Because when it comes to breastfeeding, there can be a lot of roadblocks, sadly more than you might expect. One roadblock is the lack of support—the people who will judge you or question you or otherwise make you doubt yourself and your decisions. There can be physical roadblocks. And I'm sorry to say, that many—too many—breastfeeding "failures" actually fall squarely at the feet of medical professionals. And so, here I'll address the soon-after-birth medical obstacles, or those obstacles too often placed in the way of new nursing mothers by well-meaning medical professionals. (Part Two helps guide new moms through the other medical obstacles—nipple pain, low milk supply, oversupply—as well as some of the social and emotional issues.

A FEW OF THE ROADBLOCKS TO ESTABLISHING A SUCCESSFUL BREASTFEEDING RELATIONSHIP

EMOTIONAL: You don't have the support you need. If this is the case, it's truly up to you to find support. Your hospital almost certainly has a breastfeeding support group meeting down the hallway right now. Or contact La Leche League and go to a few meetings. Seek out someone who supports and understands. Then pay it forward.

MEDICAL (related to your baby): These are the ones addressed directly in this chapter. The most common reasons doctors give to supplement are what I've termed the Three Bs, and I'll describe them each in more depth as we continue—bilirubin levels, blood sugar levels, and birthweight changes. We'll also see why "just one bottle" can be harmful, not just from a psychological perspective, but from a medical one as well.

PHYSICAL (related to you and your body): Nipple pain, I'll talk about it briefly here because it is the most common physical barrier for women breastfeeding in the early days, and I'll address it more in-depth in the question-and-answers in Chapter 10. It's actually not as common as you may believe for women to be physically incapable of producing enough milk, though I'll address that specifically in Chapter 9. I'll also talk about the flip side, which also interferes with a successful breastfeeding relationship, of over-production, as well as the much more common *perception* that you aren't producing enough milk.

THE THREE BS: BILIRUBIN, BLOOD SUGAR, AND BIRTHWEIGHT

Remember how I mentioned that we medical professionals are often the ones who undermine the breastfeeding relationship? I want to look at that in much more depth here, explaining the reasons doctors do sometimes recommend supplementing, and when it makes sense to do so (and when the numbers don't mean as much as the doctors may think). In my experience, the number one reason for new breastfeeding moms to be told to supplement is one of the Three Bs, and I'll take a look at each of them in order in the sections that follow: bilirubin, blood sugar, and birthweight. (Oh, and I'll throw a surprise fourth B in there later, just because I'm me and that sounds like fun.)

BILIRUBIN: OR YELLOW IS JUST A COLOR

Ah yes, the Three Bs—blood sugar, birthweight, and bilirubin. I'm going to start with my favorite—bilirubin. In other words, this section is about jaundice.

This topic had been in the background of my thoughts, a question I'd been struggling with in regard to its impact on breastfeeding, when I took a review course for my medical boards. Yes, there was a question about jaundice. And the answer—the answer termed the "correct answer"—was to supplement a healthy baby with formula. And that bummed me out.

Jaundice is a color. Yellow to be exact. It appears in nearly every newborn. Something that appears in nearly every newborn is normal.

The yellow pigment comes from bilirubin, which is, in turn, found inside red blood cells. In the womb, the baby's lungs are the placenta. The placenta is not very good at air exchange, so the baby, to compensate, makes lots of red blood cells to carry oxygen. When the baby is born, he doesn't need the red blood cells. They are destroyed, releasing bilirubin, making the baby yellow.

Waste not, want not.

Bilirubin appears to be an antioxidant. You get antioxidants from your diet, but a baby doesn't take in much volume, so the bilirubin serves as an antioxidant source until the baby can get enough from his diet.

There are times when yellow is a problem. Like when you aren't a newborn or you are a premie. Or when your baby's blood type doesn't match yours. The challenge for providers is to distinguish which children are at risk for complications from the increased bilirubin load. In order to decide what interventions, if any, are needed, we need to consider the age of the infant, the timing of the jaundice, the level of the serum bilirubin, and how the kids are eating. (I threw that last one in there since the AAP policy on jaundice doesn't mention it at all in their policy statement.) But, in general, healthy, term newborns turn yellow. It is not a disease—it's a color.

And while I've mentioned the level of the bilirubin, notice that it's in the context of the gestational and the chronological age of the baby, the timing of the jaundice, and (by my addition) how well the baby is transferring breastmilk.

I had this fabulously scarring episode when I was a very tired resident where I mentioned that a child's white blood cell count was 13.5 (yes, I still remember that number). My attending physician stopped me, wrote 13.5 on a piece of paper, and threw it into the air. When it landed at my feet, he said, "Jenny, what's that?"

I dutifully replied, "It's this child's white blood cell count."

He then uttered words that have stuck with me forever, "No, it's a random number flying through the air."

In other words, the level of bilirubin can't be interpreted without knowing more about the baby.

Let's try a case. (I wrote this one for the AAP Breastfeeding Curriculum.) The patient is a three-day-old exclusively breastfed girl, born at term after an induced vaginal delivery. The baby nursed well in the delivery room within an hour after delivery and has been skin-to-skin with mom. She has been feeding every three hours since. The baby's last stool, about 18 hours ago, was black and tarry. The baby and mother have the same blood type. A bedside transcutaneous bilirubin measurement at 24 hours of age places the baby in the "high intermediate" range.

Mother's concerns:

- Her nipples are cracked and bleeding.

- Her breasts are soft, and it doesn't seem as though her milk has "come in" yet.

- The baby has lost weight.

- The baby does not seem as alert as she was the day before.

What Factors May Be Contributing to the Baby's Hyperbilirubinemia?

Healthy breastfed infants normally have increased, non-pathologic elevations in serum bilirubin, sometimes called "breastmilk jaundice." Breastmilk jaundice can last for weeks and is thought to be beneficial to the infants because bilirubin is an antioxidant. This is important because, as I mentioned above, newborns do not have other sources of antioxidants.

Breastmilk jaundice needs to be distinguished from "starvation jaundice," which may indicate a pathologic condition. One of these conditions is decreased caloric intake, and in our case, this caloric deprivation is likely secondary to a breastfeeding problem.

This baby girl is likely to have starvation jaundice because of poor milk transfer. Nipple trauma is caused by a poor latch. If the baby is latched incorrectly, she cannot transfer milk and will not get the calories needed to facilitate the excretion of bilirubin. Another indication of poor milk transfer is the presence of black, tarry meconium stool at day of life three. Colostrum, the first milk made for the baby, is a laxative that promotes the excretion of meconium. In general, meconium should be well past dark and tarry by this point. (And, as you know, I really dislike the term "milk coming in." It's been there all along. Just a different recipe!)

What Does It Mean to Be in the "High Intermediate" Range?

The American Academy of Pediatrics recommends performing an assessment of every infant for the risk of severe hyperbilirubinemia. Transcutaneous bilirubin levels are a way to estimate the serum bilirubin level. Once obtained, that level is plotted on a nomogram (sometimes referred to as the "Bhutani curve") according to the baby's age in hours. The nomogram is divided into risk levels. "High Intermediate" risk means the baby has a high intermediate risk of a subsequent bilirubin level exceeding the 95th percentile. It means the baby has a high intermediate risk of the bilirubin getting higher. The magic number where danger occurs is not known.

The goal of the measurement and subsequent graph plotting is to prevent kernicterus, a totally preventable, devastating neurologic disease. Nothing about checking levels and graph plotting involves "assessing a feeding." We should work on getting that in there.

While this screening can identify babies at risk for severe hyperbilirubinemia, it does not predict the risk of kernicterus or other complications of severe hyperbilirubinemia. Again, the "curve" does not predict the risk of kernicterus. It predicts who is at risk for the bilirubin getting higher. No screening test currently exists that will reliably identify all infants at risk of developing kernicterus. Most children are not at risk for the development of kernicterus and not all children with kernicterus have a history of hyperbilirubinemia. (Makes you wonder why we screen... sorry, soap box.)

What Do We Do Next?

Since the cause of the baby's jaundice is likely "starvation jaundice," we need to increase the baby's caloric intake. **We need to feed the baby.** We need to evaluate the latch or enlist the help of someone, such as a lactation consultant, who can help this mother breastfeed without pain. If the baby needs to be supplemented, our first choice is her mother's expressed breastmilk, so we need to supply mom with a pump and show her how to appropriately use it.

For management of subsequent bilirubin levels, we can follow the AAP policy statement on "Management of Hyperbilirubinemia in the Newborn Infant 35 or More Weeks of Gestation."

The important message here is that poor management of breastfeeding is an important cause of neonatal jaundice and every effort should be made to facilitate early breastfeeding success.

Blood Sugars: Or Random Numbers Flying Through the Air, Part 2

Next up on my parade of Bs—blood sugar. As you'll recall from the previous section where I told my attending physician a patient's white cell count was 13.5 and he threw the paper in the air saying, "it's a random number flying through the air." Guess what? I'm going to continue on this theme—of random numbers flying through the air—as we ponder blood sugar (glucose) screening.

First, what's supposed to happen? What's normal? Well, a healthy, full-term infant, delivered vaginally, comes into the world, and all sorts of amazing, hardwired things happen. We talked about this is in the "Normal Newborn," so let's just focus on blood sugar.

In a healthy, full-term infant, the blood sugar normally drops, and then recovers without intervention in a couple of hours. The blood sugar recovers through the pathways that create usable sources of energy, mostly for the brain. In newborns, glucose is not the only source of energy. Glucose and ketone formation (and some other alternate body "fuels") work together to make sure the newborn brain does not suffer injury.

This is supposed to happen. This is normal. The baby goes from the placenta-driven world to the real world and has to adapt. The breastfed term newborn has lower blood sugars, but higher levels of ketones and other fuels to keep the baby going than formula-fed kids. Breastfeed babies are normal. Therefore, this drop in blood sugar that the baby makes up for with ketone bodies is normal.

Since we measure blood glucose and not blood glucose plus ketone-fuel-things-that-make-your-brain-happy, we get a number. A number that tells us glucose levels, but doesn't measure alternative sources of energy—a random number flying through the air.

So, let's say we get a baby who has a measured glucose of 25. Well? Now what?

Does that baby have symptoms? If not, why did we check her glucose level? Kids without symptoms are doing something right. Why would we "fix" that? A glucose of 25 may mean nothing if the baby makes up for it with creation of alternative fuels, which they do normally, and which we don't check when we measure "blood sugar." Kids with no symptoms from their low blood sugar don't need to be treated. The answer is to do what we should be doing already—skin-to-skin snuggling, feeding within an hour after delivery, and frequent breastfeeding, since breastfeeding is a source of sugar. You can continue to check blood sugars until they are normal, however you define normal, and if you checked blood sugars to begin with.

When we treat symptom-less blood sugar with something other than breastmilk, the production of alternative fuels gets messed up. Low blood sugar drove those pathways to create alternative fuel production. When we give formula or glucose water, we don't need other ways of finding sugar—it's right there, and those other newborn pathways may be delayed in working. We messed with physiology. That wasn't nice because now, without those helping pathways, the kids may need continued supplements.

A baby with a low blood sugar and symptoms, well, that's a problem. Symptomatic blood sugar can show up as irritability, seizures, lethargy, turning blue, coma, not being able to maintain temperature, and irregular breathing, among other evil things. Now look at that list and see if we want to chalk any one of those symptoms up to just a low blood sugar. That baby could be sick. Really sick. Like "take them to the ICU sick."

What's up with that baby that they didn't compensate for their low glucose with ketone bodies? What went wrong? Maybe the baby is a premie and can't create ketone bodies or alternative body fuel. Maybe the baby is simply cold and should be snuggling on mom's chest. Or maybe that baby has overwhelming infection, congenital heart disease, lung disease, liver disease, or is otherwise really sick. Kids with low blood sugar and symptoms can have awful neurological problems. Why, though? Because of the blood sugar itself or because of the underlying reason the baby couldn't make up for that normal drop in blood sugar?

So...low blood sugar with no symptoms. Not an issue.

Breastmilk meets the nutritional requirements of healthy, term infants, and those same healthy, term, exclusively breastfed infants do not develop symptomatic low blood sugar because they are not eating. Healthy term infants do not need to have their blood sugar screened.

BUT...low blood sugar with symptoms: Big problem.

These children have some reason they can't make up for low blood sugar with other fuels. They may be, among other things, premature, small for gestational age, an infant of a diabetic mother (especially if the diabetes was poorly controlled), sick, or withdrawing from a substance mom was taking. These kids should be screened. Because then, the number means something.

Birthweight: Or I'm Sure I Saw That Baby on a Treadmill

I've been calling bilirubin, birthweight, and blood sugars my "Three Bs" and have been discussing them as "random numbers flying through the air." This birthweight thing is a sticky issue for me because when my third son was born (yes, to my board-certified pediatrician, IBCLC self) and I was told he had lost 10% of his birthweight, at midnight no less, I burst into tears. And for that time, my confidence was shot.

But a more rational me, with the sun out the following day, realized that I was a giant water balloon when my son was born, he looked a little puffy, and I'm pretty sure you can't really lose 10 percent of your birthweight in a day or two unless you are pooping and puking your brains out, or maybe you're exercising, or you are exercising while pooping and puking. I've seen some things in nurseries that make me go "hmmmm," but I'm pretty sure I've never seen a gym. Maybe I'm not that observant.

But I did a little, unscientific sampling of wise people on our Lakeshore Breastfeeding Medicine page on Facebook, and I heard a few things repeatedly—you can get a bunch of IV fluids during delivery that may, if the placenta is still hooked up, transfer to the baby, making both you and the baby water-logged, and using the same scale to weigh the baby makes intuitive sense. Of course, nobody bought into my treadmill theory.

I also read lots of opinions about "not having any milk yet." We need to tackle this issue because that line of thinking may lead to buy-in that this weight loss is clinically significant, and you can't provide for your baby. I

want to make sure I'm clear here: I'm talking about the first days. If the baby is down 10 percent from birthweight at day six, we have a problem. But the idea that the "milk isn't in yet" needs to be addressed. Your milk is in. Colostrum, while it may be a different recipe from the subsequent milk you make, is still precious, valuable, and perfect.

"He isn't getting anything" or "I can't satisfying him" are said way too often. Understanding what newborns do is critical to believing your body can feed that beautiful new baby you just introduced to the world.

So why is this a problem? Kids are getting supplemented. Sometimes without or against parental informed consent. As we've already seen, 'just one bottle" can make a huge difference in how a baby's immune system develops. We should have a very good reason for supplementing. But do we?

Check this out from the CDC: According to this graph, about 20 percent of kids in the U.S. are being supplemented with formula before two days of age. That makes no sense. And it's heartbreaking, confidence-rotting, and is probably due to the Three Bs and random numbers flying through the air.

So why would we supplement? According to the Academy of Breastfeeding Medicine's Protocol number three on supplementation, we would supplement for:

- Maternal illness resulting in separation of infant and mother

- Infant with inborn error of metabolism (galactosemia)

- Infant who is unable to feed at the breast (congenital malformation, illness)

- Maternal medication contraindicated in breastfeeding

- Breast pathology or prior breast surgery resulting in poor milk production

- Intolerable pain during feeding unrelieved by interventions

- Significant dehydration—clinical and laboratory evidence that is not improved with skilled assessment and proper management of breastfeeding

- Delayed bowel movements or meconium stools on day five

- Insufficient intake despite an adequate milk supply (poor milk transfer)

- Hyperbilirubinemia, which might be associated with starvation, as in "lack-of – breastmilk" jaundice.

And we would choose to supplement first with expressed human milk, donor milk, and if necessary infant formula.

We wouldn't supplement for:

- Sleepy infant with fewer than eight to 12 feedings in the first 24-48 hours with less than seven percent weight loss and no sign of illness.

- Bilirubin levels less than 18 after 72 hours of age when the baby is feeding well and stooling, and the weight loss is less than seven percent.

- The infant who is fussy at night or constantly feeding for several hours.

- The tired or sleeping mother.

Where does the seven percent come from? When I have asked, the only answer I've received is that it's "just standard." But it's a number. What else should we check? Well, I like poop. Colostrum is a great laxative, the more poop, the more milk we know is being transferred. Maybe we could look at the rate of the decline of the weight loss. Did the baby lose seven percent night one, 1.5 percent night two, and one percent night three? That might be an indicator that the baby lost its water-balloon status and is improving. Maybe we could have someone who knows what they are doing help the mother (education, education, education...). Maybe we could empower the mother how to interpret the weight loss that may happen after an induction, epidural, and then C-section, and getting nine gallons of fluid (ok, slight exaggeration). Empowering the mother and her support system with knowledge about what is normal and expected is crucial.

Numbers need to be interpreted in the context of the mom, baby, birth, and the breastfeeding situation or they are worthless.

Nipple Pain: Look at the Latch First

Nipple pain is no small problem, so I'm going to take one look at it here as we address obstacles in the first days of breastfeeding. I'll also examine the issue in more depth in Chapter 10.

The thing is, pain is a powerful motivator to quit breastfeeding, to quit anything, and I get that. That's why it's so important for me to emphasize:

Pain means something is wrong. And here's something else I know, many new mothers describe that pain right from the first feeding. Many more experience it in the first week. And many of these moms don't seek help and instead wean.

We know from research and from practical experience that proper positioning and an appropriate latch can save your nursing experience. What do you need to know about the latch?

A good latch doesn't compress the nipple. If your baby comes off the breast and the nipple is compressed (like a new lipstick), then we know the tongue was in the wrong spot, touching the nipple and causing trauma. That trauma, if it continues, can lead to worsening sores and may be a jumping off point for infection.

There is a long list of other things that can cause pain besides a poor latch (and resulting infection). Breast engorgement. Baby tongue-tie. Certain medical conditions. See Chapter 10 for more on this.

But for now, it's important to emphasize: Pain is not normal, so something is wrong. And the first ten reasons on the list of why nipples might be sore is a poor latch. As I may have said a million times before, the latch should not be painful, so finding a resource who is specifically knowledgeable about assessing a latch is really, really important. Remember: No one can say from looking at the latch from outside whether or not it is "right."

Pain is a tiger. Don't let anyone tell you it is normal, to be expected, or all part of the breastfeeding deal.

Now, whether it's because of one of the three Bs, because of nipple pain or another medical obstacle, or simply because a well-meaning someone is urging you to get some sleep while you can, you may encounter another obstacle in those first days right after you give birth the one I call the "Just One Bottle syndrome." Sound harmless? Let's take a look.

"Just One Bottle" and Its Impact on Your Baby's Gut and Immune System

So here we are. Your baby has been born. She has gone directly to your chest, found your nipple, perhaps been nourished by colostrum. All is well. And yet, you may hear someone urging you to give your newborn "just one bottle," perhaps so you can rest, or perhaps... well there are all sorts of possible reasons. "Just one bottle," they may say. "What harm could it do?"

Well, let's take a look at that, a geeky, medical look at good bacteria, the role of breastmilk in immune system development, and that "just one" bottle. (And yes, I will warn you that the pages that follow are indeed filled with somewhat complicated medical terms and information... and I promise those of you who hate that sort of thing that I will "sum it up" again at the end with a friendlier, less intense version.)

Ready to go back with me now to that perfect world in which a full-term, healthy newborn comes into the world vaginally... Again, I want to talk about normal. I do know the process doesn't go normally all the time. And yet, I want to emphasize that the delivery of the baby vaginally—in other words, close to the anus—is critical for immune system development. The healthy, term newborn's gut is sterile (without bacteria), and the bacteria that get into that perfect, pristine newborn gut are truly important. During a vaginal delivery, the largely harmless bacteria around the mother's anus are the bacteria getting into the newborn gut. They increase in number, compete for food and space, and help coordinate efforts to create a healthy gut for the baby. With the exception of our skin, the gut is the largest immune system organ in our body.

Because breastfeeding is normal, what happens to healthy, term newborns who are breastfed is normal. The newborn has a delay in their immune response to bacteria. A delay? To a bacteria? Yup. Normal. After delivery, the newborn gut has many challenges from invaders that may not be friendly. Doesn't seem too smart not to fight back.

We all have mechanisms in our body to fight infection. In the gut it's called Gut Associated Lymphoid Tissue (GALT), and it's ready to roll at 19 weeks of gestation. All of the things that make up the GALT are waiting for a specific series of events to occur after delivery, when, if it proceeds normally, will result in a functioning immune system.

The sequence of those events is important. For example, after the good (commensal) bacteria has set up shop in the newborn gut, something called an "isolated lymphoid follicle" in the intestine of the baby develops. It's activated by substances in colostrum and helps with T-cell development and function.

T-cells are part of what is called the "innate" system. They mature in the thymus, an immune system structure found in the neck and chest of newborns. Human milk activates resting thymus cells, helping to shape the immune function of these cells. Breastfed kids have a larger thymus than those that are not breastfed; the thymus of the breastfed child is up to twice the size of a child not breastfed. The innate immune system contains cells that kill bacteria, but they do it by also causing inflammation and tissue damage.

The innate immune system is different from the "adaptive" immune system, which is very specific to certain invaders. (Never being very good at immunology, but being really great at American football, I see the innate system as the offensive line, generally protecting the quarterback. The adaptive immune system is more like the wide receiver or cornerback—a player with a more specific job.)

The cells of the adaptive immune system, antibodies, come in several flavors: Immunoglobulin M (IgM), which is the first type of antibody produced and isn't very specific; IgG, which is transferred across the placenta and is the only immunoglobulin that the baby gets from mom and has at birth (the newborn, with only IgG is essentially immuno-compromised); IgE, which isn't too relevant here; and IgA which rocks. IgA is a "sticky" immunoglobulin that protects surface areas from infection. A special type of IgA, secretory IgA, is found in huge numbers in human milk and protects the airway, gut, and other mucous membranes from infection.

So, we have a new baby exposed immediately to bacteria...why no inflammation? Well, the activity of the T-cells is delayed for about 10 days (remember, T-cells cause inflammation and tissue damage) and secretory IgA helps. It's made by mom in response to infections in her environment and passed to the baby through breastfeeding. Moms and babies should stay together. This is one good reason—mom can't make antibodies to things that the baby is exposed to if the baby isn't with her.

Human milk (i.e., breastmilk) also contains special sugars, oligosaccharides, which help feed good bacteria. In fact, they are necessary for the good bacteria to grow. Plus, they are a type of prebiotic—something that can block bad bacteria before they ever get to the surface of the gut. They let the probiotics, the good bacteria, stay in the gut. And because they never let the bad bacteria get to the gut surface, no innate immune system is needed, and we get no inflammation or tissue damage. Oligosaccharides also work with certain receptors (called Toll-Like Receptors). These receptors work in the first five days (when are our kids getting supplemented?) and are controlled tightly—like hour by hour.

In the time that the immune system is delayed, oligosaccharides, toll like receptors, and good bacteria protect against bad bacteria and avoid the need for an inflammatory response. Any alteration in human milk or addition of formula interferes with toll-like receptor function, changes the bacteria that the baby's gut gets exposed to, and can then lead to inflammation and tissue damage, the result we are trying so hard to avoid.

The lesson? Let's make sure we know why we are supplementing. And know the real implications of "just one bottle."

(If you're a geeky, science medicine type like myself and interested in more detailed information on this topic, I'd suggest a very nice book from Dr. Lars Hanson entitled *Immunobiology of Human Milk*.)

Thoughts About Running (Or a Thinly Veiled Metaphor About Breastfeeding)

As we end this chapter about all the obstacles you may face as a breastfeeding mom—about the roadblocks put in your way, even by well-meaning medical professions—I'd like to talk about running again. This time, I'm thinking more about the runs that are difficult—difficult to even start, but that become so much more than just a run, when you have people around to support you. And so, my thoughts on just such a run:

I run starting at my house because I live across the street from a beautiful state park. I've been running races in that park since I was small. I biked the trails with good friends when I was in high school. I bought my house partly because I thought it would be awesome to get on those trails whenever I wanted. Nearly every trail turn is associated with some memory—good and bad. I know the exact place where I decided I needed to quit my former job, where I found my dad after he had fallen from his bike, and where my dad found me when I was on a long run and decided to run with me, helping me finish a 10-miler I never would have finished otherwise. I know the spot in the park's half-marathon course where my brother and his friend joined me and helped me get control of my form and breathing, and provided such encouragement that I finished, when I thought I couldn't take another step.

And I know the terrain. I know where the hills are, the uneven pavement, the blind curves, the places that are going to hurt as I run them, and the places where I can recover. No matter how good I'm feeling, how good I think my form and breathing are, I can start to feel the seeds of previous pain. And sometimes I get lucky and know that I have successfully beaten that hill or that stretch of pavement, and I get a second wind. But I can get ready for those hard places, especially the hills, ages before I even get close. By the time I get there, I've convinced myself that hill is Mt. Kilimanjaro.

My run today was tough. It's hot. My knee is in a brace. But there's not a cloud in the sky and I just can't pass days like these by when four months from now I may be running in snow pants. Plus, if there's a harder way to do something, I must do it that way. I know and accept that about myself. I ran without my Garmin or my iPod. I needed to do that today—just me and the messages from my body.

I picked a trail I run that has a few big hills, and I felt myself getting ready for Mt. Kilimanjaro before I took my first step. Bad sign...expecting pain and failure before I even start. So I tried visualizing success. Sometimes I picture running with helium balloons on my back, helping me up the hill. Today, I saw my friends, with their kids, holding a sign that said "You run like a Kenyan" (a personal favorite of mine I saw during a half-marathon in Indianapolis). My friends were jumping up and down and cheering me on. And a few were stepping in front of the parts of my imaginary crowd that weren't cheering. As I visualized them, I got control of my pace, picked up my head, and felt more confident. I saw them at every tough curve. By the time I got back to my house, to what I intended to be my finish line, I kept going.

So thanks to my twitter pals at #momrun for helping me finish my run feeling good. For holding the sign, for protecting me from the people who won't cheer. You are awesome and everyone should have someone like you, to make you feel like a Kenyan. And to love, praise, and respect you, even on days when you just can't climb Mt. Kilimanjaro.

So step five: Know that not every step is going to be easy. Be prepared for the roadblocks. Have a plan for getting around them. And, hopefully, enlist support. It might not be simple, but you can get through.

CHAPTER 6.
WHEN IN NEED,
TELL YOUR STORY.

Another phrase I hear too often from struggling moms is this, *"I know you're going to be mad when I tell you this, but..."* Stop! I know I've said this before, but it's so important: We moms have given away a lot of what "mothering" is to experts and books. And we need to take that power back. This isn't about what I want for your baby, or what any other healthcare provider wants for your family. It's about you and your family.

Here's the thing, we doctors are the hired help. We are the people that you and your family have chosen to help you through this journey. It's not about our judgment, or what might make us "mad." We are not the arbiters of right or wrong, good or bad. We are the people who are supposed to give you the information you need to make an informed decision, to help aid in the encouragement of and confidence in parenting instinct.

So much of what I see as a healthcare provider, so much of the advice I see being given, is counter to maternal instinct, which makes me sad to my soul. Here is what I know: If there truly were a "right" and a "wrong" way to parent, maybe six of us would make it to adulthood, and that's not good for a species that wishes to continue to exist.

My first day of medical school, one of my deans told my class, "Fifty percent of what we are teaching you is wrong. We just don't know which 50 percent." That admission has stuck with me when I begin to feel like I have it "right" or I know what is "best" for a child in my practice. It keeps me humble and open to change. All we can do as providers is give the information or make a recommendation (not make a command) based on our current knowledge base and be willing to learn and adapt when the 50 percent starts to change. I hope you, as parents, are then enabled to integrate that advice into what works for you as a family.

I am a big fan of giving messages that make sense to a family, of encouraging the course of action you already have chosen (as long as it doesn't involve juggling chain saws near the kids or parenting while on heroin, or something else we can be pretty sure is going to stay a non-recommended parenting practice!). I can't and shouldn't dictate a course of action or stifle a dialogue on topics where we might have differing opinions. In the end, as long as the debated parenting practice is not illegal, I am the paid employee. If that kind of dialogue is not encouraged, if that freedom to parent is somehow curbed by a provider who is sure they have it right, if as a mother, you feel as if you somehow have to modify what you say or outright lie about how you parent for fear of backlash from a physician, your family should fire that provider and hire a new, more compatible employee.

If you are stuck with only one doctor on the planet, then well, you should speak up. (I'll talk more about this in the third section of this book, about advocating for breastfeeding moms.) Please, take the power of motherhood back. It is yours. And you need to hold on to it.

So step six, I hope, is simple. When you need help, don't be afraid to tell your story. There's no reason to hide the truth, to modify your intentions to fit someone else's story. Take the power that is yours. And ask for help based on what you're doing and what you need.

CHAPTER 7.
ENJOY THE GOOD TIMES AND CELEBRATE EVERY STEP

The good times? Ah, these can be hard to imagine when you're, uhm, for example, locked in the bathroom, hiding from your newborn baby. Or yes, at least, that's really where I found myself in the early days of mothering and breastfeeding my third-born son.

"I will not!" I screamed at my husband. "I will not do this anymore! It hurts. This sucks. I quit!"

"Honey, you know you can't do that," he responded in his psychiatrist voice.

The stupid latch. How many had I fixed? How many mothers in exactly my spot had I helped? And here I was, pediatrician, lactation consultant, hiding in my bathroom, hiding from the latch and my baby. My baby boy, who looked just like his dad, the one making sense when I just wanted to cry.

"Fine. I won't quit" I sniveled. "But I promise I won't like it."

And you know what? I broke that promise. It took a while, yes, but once I got past the pain and the difficulties, and all the mess that seems to consume our lives in those early, long days of breastfeeding a newborn, well, eventually I did like breastfeeding again.

And, I'm pretty sure, you'll reach that point, too. Some of us sooner than others (and some of us sooner with some of our babies than with others). But you'll reach the point when you look down at that baby nursing, happy, and you'll see those chubby thighs, and you'll realize: I did that. My body did that. And these are the times to enjoy.

Because, as hard as it is to believe in those early days when every hour can seem like a lifetime, life does go on. And guess what? You're a part of it again!

So what can you expect now that you're hitting your stride, now that things are looking good? What might change? Well, as your baby gets more interested in the outside world, she may start getting distracted while feeding. Older babies turn their heads to watch siblings or other new things in their ever-expanding worlds. Sometimes, they don't have the courtesy to release the nipple (ouch!) as they explore. Sometimes, it's like holding onto a trapeze artist. You may find nursing in a darker, less stimulating place may curb that behavior. (Or you may just find it cute. The first couple of times I got a foot in the face or my son wanted to watch the world, hold onto one breast, and nurse from the other, I found it fun and sort of fascinating. The first few times.)

You may be headed back to work. If it helps your transition, I only cried for the first seven weeks I went back to work after my oldest son was born. But that was before all the new workplace protections were put into place in the United States. Section 4207 of the *Patient Protection and Affordable Care Act* (also known as Healthcare Reform) states that employers shall provide breastfeeding employees with "reasonable break time" and a private, non-bathroom place to express breastmilk during the workday, up until the child's first birthday. Those companies with more than 50 employees are required to do this. Those with less than 50 have to apply for a "hardship exemption." And the "Business Case for Breastfeeding" (www.ask.hrsa.gov) can also help make that transition easier. Easier, hopefully, than seven weeks of crying.

You may also be looking forward to starting complementary foods, meaning something other than breastmilk. There is consensus now by every important group who weighs in on these things that exclusive breastmilk feedings is what we want for the first six months. I know that's practically heresy in a culture so used to feeding kids when they are just a few weeks or months old. So when we decide that the kids are ready for food, what food do we start with? The American tradition has always been rice cereal. In Germany, many kids start with carrots or cooked pumpkin. In Holland they start with bananas or apple mash. There are no studies out there that tell us what the best foods to start with are. Which means that the insistence on cereal in our kids' diet is a *tradition*, not a *necessity*. In fact, the AAP has officially stated that we need to "throw out the rice cereal."

Okay, we'll get to all of that. But first—you know how I feel about these sleep issues—we have to tackle that question you're sure to face, perhaps even on your first day back at work, or on the playground, or at the holiday gatherings with your "older" nursing baby.

Sleep—Part 3: Is Your Baby Sleeping Through the Night Yet?

The answer is almost always "no," but when we give that answer, we feel like bad parents, and we start to believe that something is wrong with our child...as if normal babies were never meant to be held all the time and were meant to sleep all by themselves!

Here's something I've noticed: We spend so much time dreaming of what our children will be and very little time realizing what they are. Let's say, for the sake of argument, that human evolution is like a football field. Human beings as a genus start at the far end of the field, and we, as a species, show up at about the opposite 10-yard line. At about the one-inch line (and that's generous), we, as an industrial society, show up. Why am I rambling about this? Because we have to understand that the way we do things is a new idea...but the babies we bring into this world don't know about the way we do things. They are programmed to do things that normal, vulnerable human babies have been doing for thousands of years.

And, as I've mentioned before, human babies are really vulnerable. Remember: Our babies arrive in the world as the most neurologically immature primate of them all, and remain the most dependent on a caregiver for the longest period of time. Our kids can't keep themselves warm, get food, walk, speak, or reason. They need to be near mom during sleep for a reason: this immature baby, with little in the way of self-preservation skills, needs to hang out with the source of food and warmth, with the person who is most likely to wake up to meet the needs they express in the middle of the night.

Okay, I already know this about newborns so many parents say to me. But they add, *"My baby is now (eight weeks) (ten weeks) (three months) old. Shouldn't she be sleeping thought the night yet?"* The answer isn't much different. Older infants get up at night, but less often. It is normal even for one-year-olds to not be sleeping through the night.

How about this idea that we have to teach our kids to "soothe" themselves? I would argue that a several-month-old child is still not able to feed themselves, find food, or do any other thing that it would take to live independently. How could they soothe themselves? Soothing yourself is a complex emotional task, hardly one that we would expect from a creature who can't walk or talk. They are speaking up because they need something. If they need something, even if it just to feel safe, why shouldn't we help them? And imagine this—you are up crying at night and the person you love decides to ignore you. What might happen the next morning? What might happen is that person continues to ignore your cries for help and comfort?

And so this brings us all back to the topic of sleeping arrangements. The choice of where our children sleep affects (and there is research to show all of this): breastfeeding duration, feeding frequency, infant sleep position, arousal patterns, temperature, carbon dioxide levels, crying, heart rate, and parental emotional expectations.

Babies who have more skin-to-skin contact with their parents show better oxygen delivery, less frequent crying, higher temperatures, better weight gain, better digestion, and less physiologic markers of infant stress. (It's why kids who are held more have less colic.) So based on that, it makes sense that more contact with mom and dad makes for a more physiologically sound child.

So the question now goes, *"How come my friend's baby sleeps through the night?"* The answer? I don't know. I don't even know what that means. When

I ask about what that means, I get a great variety of answers. Some people think six hours of sleep at night is "through the night," other people want to sleep like they did before they had kids. I would guess that the kids aren't sleeping through the night, but that the implications of admitting that your kid isn't sleeping are too nasty to admit. We equate "good sleepers" with good kids and "bad sleepers" with bad kids. Really, we make moral implications from normal baby behaviors. And of course, parents of good sleepers are good parents.

Plus, feeding choice plays a role here. Formula-fed kids sleep differently than breastfed kids. Formula-fed kids sleep for longer stretches of time and, therefore, have less contact with their parents at night. Formula-fed children are much more likely to be sleeping alone.

The sleep training techniques that have been sold in the U.S. have never been shown to be associated with anything good for infants, but it has been associated with bad stuff, like more anxious children and behavior disturbances. There is no emotional, social, or intellectual benefit to the kids, nor has it ever been shown to help us develop into healthy adult sleepers.

So...we have to decide what we want from our kids sleeping through the night. I would guess that all the good things that we want for our kids' futures mean that we don't have them sleep through the night. And so, my favorite answer to the question, "Is your baby sleeping through the night yet?" is "She's sleeping like a baby!" Yes, let your baby be a baby.

THE ONE-YEAR MARK: CELEBRATING THE JOURNEY

"It showed me that I did and was doing something special and that is worth recognition. It also made me want to continue."

"It was a huge congratulations for us, and it made the kids excited that we'd done a good thing together. It showed others that you supported us through our struggles, which I think is HUGE to advertise, explain, and share with other Moms who want to nurse."

"For me it was a finish line. A goal to make it to. Thank you for that, cause I would have quit sooner."

These are quotes from mothers in my practice, and they are talking, simply, about a t-shirt.

I give a t-shirt that reads "Got Breastmilk?" to breastfeeding moms and their one-year-olds at the one-year well visit. I've been doing it for years. I pay for the shirts myself, and I do it because I figure that if you make it through all the obstacles that we throw in the way of successful breastfeeding, somebody should congratulate you.

"The shirts represented that I had done something really important for my kids. I was thrilled to earn one for both kids. I also wanted to show others that active moms do breastfeed."

I have heard courageous stories of breastfeeding against overwhelming obstacles and am always impressed with the determination of mothers to continue past those obstacles. I have also heard the pain when mothers don't meet their nursing goals.

So we celebrate the journey. We don't need to devalue the breastfeeding experience or breastfeeding itself; we need to celebrate the success, and then transition to the next steps in parenting.

I have thought about doing this giveaway at different times in the experience or giving these t-shirts to celebrate special achievements prior to a year, but the thing is, I like the idea of having these shirts on one-year-olds, instead of babies, as a way of demonstrating that nursing a toddler is still normal.

"It was a great bonding experience and I loved every minute of it. It was great to know I could breastfeed for that long and not feel ashamed like some people think it is out there in the world."

"A special 'thank you' to you...for keeping me motivated through the (occasional) physical pain, for the words of encouragement on those days when I just wanted my body back, and for arming me with the confidence and intellectual, fact-based fire-power to defend my decision against those, "You're STILL breastfeeding?" people!"

We all measure success differently. It could be that mom decided to breastfeed at all. It could be that she achieved her own goals. Sometimes, I think the mother just needs a cheerleader to help to her continue to meet her goals. Who would have thought a shirt could do it?

"There were times, around ten months, where I was ready to stop, but knowing that (my daughter) could have a t-shirt, however silly that is, was a big deal for me. Once I hit that year mark, it was easy to continue."

"That darn shirt kept me going on the days I wanted to give up."

"I didn't think I would make it, especially working full time, but I needed the t-shirt! Before I knew it, he was 16 months and still nursing, even with a brother well on the way!"

"Knowing that I had overcome a lot of obstacles and trying times to achieve something great for my child. The t-shirt, although nothing huge like a trip to Disney world, shows to everyone what you and your child have accomplished."

I'm sure there are a myriad of reasons why the mothers in my practice chose to continue nursing, but I'm glad there are some women I could help reach or exceed their breastfeeding goals with a little recognition and an acknowledgment of their journey.

And that journey, I'd like to point out, does not need to end at the one-year mark. Which brings us to another journey to celebrate—those who breastfeed past a year and even well into (and beyond) toddlerhood, and why they need special support.

When Breastmilk Turns to Water and Everyone Says a Cow Makes Better Milk Than You Do

I really do think that if you nurse for a year someone should have a party for you. The best I've been able to do is give out those t-shirts I just talked about earlier. I've given out more shirts than I can count now, and I have a (now not-so-current) recognition list of "one year" dyads on my website.

So with all these moms in my practice reaching that goal, I began to consider doing something to recognize those mothers who continued to breastfeed to 18 months. But guess what? Those wonderful moms, who took the shirt and the congrats at a year, said "no thank you" when I mentioned what I was thinking about. Why? They didn't want people to know. They'd nurse, but they didn't want public acknowledgement. They were "closet" nursers and they were okay with it.

The one-year visit is also an opportunity to talk about the benefits of continuing to nurse after a year. I'm going to try not to call it "extended breastfeeding" since that reveals a cultural bias that exists where I live, but maybe not where you do. Worldwide, nursing two to four years is just normal. And before cultural biases interrupt the discussion, the AAP policy statement on "Breastfeeding and the Use of Human Milk" says that there "is no upper limit to the duration of breastfeeding and no evidence of psychologic or developmental harm from breastfeeding into the third year of life or longer."

So what happens at a year? Well, according to popular belief, as your beautiful breastfed child is sleeping the evening before their first birthday, their world gets rocked—the next day, they will discover that breastmilk serves no purpose. We have found a cow that makes better milk than mom.

How do you make a non-verbal one-year-old understand that? They are counting on that same warmth, expression of love, and wonderful nutrition that they got the day before. What's magic about that 366th day of their life?

Now really, I know that doesn't make sense and the one-year-old is probably confused, but I know some wonderful women who believe that even if they are continuing to nurse, the child still needs supplemental cow's milk "to get enough nutrients." I may live in "America's Dairyland" where we wear cheeseheads in public, but cow's milk is for cows. And since I'm usually having this conversation at a well visit, with the child right there, I can do a reasonable job of convincing the family that my physical exam suggests their child is not a cow.

The infection-fighting properties of breastmilk are still present; lysozyme, lactoferrin, and secretory IgA are present in stable amounts. There are smaller levels of protein, calcium, and long chain fatty acids when compared to the milk of a three-month-old, but we aren't talking about a three-month-old, who is only getting breastmilk. Our toddler is getting complementary foods. Plus we know that moms who nurse longer lower their risk of breast cancer.

I get it. Many people, including most healthcare providers, don't understand why you'd want to nurse for more than a year. But they aren't the ones trying to calm a screaming 15-month-old. I'm just saying, if I had to pick between the crying kid I need to distract and make happy somehow and the crying child who I can nurse and calm and get to smile in about five minutes, I'm picking the latter.

Someday, I'll be able to do something for my friends, the closet nursers, and I'll know we're making progress in my little slice of the world. Maybe then we can convince the rest of the world that nursing a toddler is normal. Until then, I guess I'll just keep my "beyond one year" t-shirts and quietly acknowledge the closet nursers, bravely giving their children the very best they have, for as long as they both enjoy it.

THE FINAL STEPS: WEANING

Ah, the end of this journey. It's been a long road and one, I'm certain, that's taken you places you never could have imagined when you first began. And now it's time for it to be done. It's time to wean. I'll go into much more detail about how to wean in Chapter 15. For now, I'd like to just look at the why.

Ideally, when to wean is a decision that you and your child make together. Realistically, I know, as many moms head back to work, this may be hard to do. And often, there are other factors that play into your decision to wean. But before we get into any specifics, let me say that if you have been told to wean because of a medication you are taking or because of an illness, pregnancy, or surgery, double check. There's a bunch of bad information out there and lots of unnecessary weaning taking place. And if you are weaning because you've been told that breastmilk has no benefits after a certain time, just keep nursing. No formula has come close to breastmilk, and there is no cow out there making better milk for your child than you are.

Weaning is almost always accompanied by some guilt and regret. But I hope you can celebrate what you achieved and appreciate the gift you have given your child. I hope all of you know that I am really impressed with all the work you put into nursing. I have helped many moms through very difficult starts to breastfeeding, and I'm continually amazed at the motivation they have to continue to breastfeed through very difficult circumstances. Please realize that 25% of the women in the U.S. don't even try to nurse. Your kids are very lucky to have moms like you.

And so, step seven: Celebrate. Every step. Need I say more?

PART 2.
LOTS OF QUESTIONS, SOME ANSWERS, AND A FEW POSSIBLE SOLUTIONS

CHAPTER 8.
MOTHER ISSUES — GENERAL

SHOULD I GET A BREAST PUMP BEFORE MY BABY IS BORN?

Here I have to say that I sometimes think we new moms undermine ourselves by preparing a bit too much. Suddenly, there are whole lists of equipment "needs" that you're supposed to go out and buy before your baby is even born in order to *breastfeed*. Not to sound too simplistic here, but you already have pretty much all the equipment you need to breastfeed. And I've seen breast pumps actually interfere with the whole breastfeeding process, if introduced and used before you and your newborn have even had a chance to establish your breastfeeding relationship. It's mostly that whole "numbers" thing again—in this case, *how many ounces can I pump?* that really serves to undermine your own confidence. And so, in that spirit, I'll offer these suggestions on approaching breast pumps in the early days:

- If you are getting one as a shower gift, say thank you. Then lock it up to avoid temptation. :)

- If you are buying one, maybe wait until you meet your baby to see what your needs are going to be.

- But if you're a planner and having one beforehand helps, great.

- What you pump is not what the child gets and not understanding this—really and truly—is a common mistake that can undermine your efforts.

- Most hospitals will have pumps if you are separated from your baby (like for a NICU stay) or if your baby is having trouble latching, so you don't really need one in a hospital. However...

- Even the greatest electric pump stinks at getting colostrum out well. If you try to pump colostrum, hand expression is really important, too. To see it done, check out http://newborns.stanford.edu/Breastfeeding/HandExpression.html

- Your feelings about why you may want to pump may change after you meet your little one.

- Maternity leave may never be long enough, but it's still long enough to go get a pump before you go back to work.

- Bad pumping experiences can rot your confidence. That stinks.

- And the best "pump" is the one you give birth to.

WHAT FOODS SHOULD I AVOID WHILE BREASTFEEDING?

None.

Okay, well, that may not be totally true. Moms who are nursing should eat a healthy, well-balanced diet, so a diet of nothing but pork rinds and Cheetos is out. But the commonly held belief that breastfeeding moms can't have spicy foods, fatty foods, chocolate, alcoholic beverages, peanuts, cabbage, garlic, blah, blah, blah is not true.

Let's just stop and think for a bit. What do you suppose moms in Mexico, Greece, Italy, and India are eating while they are nursing? I would bet it's not boiled chicken and rice.

In fact, what mom eats flavors the breastmilk, and when the baby starts solid food, the broad exposure to flavors that they have had through breastmilk help makes the transition to solids easier and the baby's palate a little more adventurous.

Alcohol. Alcohol definitely gets into breastmilk, but it is metabolized in breastmilk as well. The level of alcohol in breastmilk is exactly the same as the level in the bloodstream at any given time. So, if you have a glass of beer and are feeling the effects of the alcohol, then don't feed the baby. If you don't feel the effects, then it's OK to nurse. There is no reason to pump and dump that milk. Strategically, it's best to nurse and then have the drink, so that by the time the baby wants to nurse again, the alcohol will have already been metabolized. Alcohol can really inhibit the let-down reflex, so be aware of that as well.

Caffeine. Caffeine also gets into milk, and because it sticks around in the body for awhile, a second cup or canned drink can have additive effects. What we are looking for is effects in the baby. If you notice that your baby is cranky after you have your triple mocha espresso, then caffeine may be a bad thing. But, as I sit here with my second can of Diet Mountain Dew, caffeine is probably okay for most nursing moms and babies.

And if you have a gassy baby? Most of the time, the diet concern is because the baby has gas. That gas can probably be fixed with a change in feeding technique (more on this in the next chapter), and really it has nothing to do with mom's diet.

Foods that may be associated with decreased milk supply: There's not a whole lot of real science behind this, but they may be worth mentioning. Sage has been used to decrease milk supply in some cultures, and I have heard that sage dressings and such (like on turkey over the holidays) can cause a dip in supply. In order for sage to cause a big drop in supply, lots has to be used, but it is a potential cause of low milk supply, so I mention it. I have heard similar things about peppermint, but I have no idea how it works.

WHAT MEDICATION CAN I TAKE WHILE I'M BREASTFEEDING?

This question can best be answered by explaining my basic principles of breastfeeding.

1. We don't throw milk away without a really, really good reason. Like you are getting chemotherapy or have decided to do heroin.

2. Most medications are compatible (I try to avoid saying "safe") with breastfeeding.

3. Most pharmacists and other health professionals don't know #1, #2, or that good pumps can be really expensive. Sometimes they give well-intentioned bad advice. Back to #1 and #2.

4. If we give it to infants, it's okay to take.

5. If you don't really need to take it (like cold medications), don't take it.

6. Most antibiotics are fine.

7. More questions? Consult Lactmed or the InfantRisk Center (www.infantrisk.com).

CAN I GET MY PERIOD WHILE I'M BREASTFEEDING?

Yes, women who breastfeed and don't use any other method of contraception don't normally ovulate, and therefore don't normally get a period in the months after they deliver. But it sometimes doesn't work that way.

Lactational Amenorrhea (no period while you are nursing) works if you nurse "intensively." The baby needs to be less than six months of age and exclusively breastfed for this method to work. "Intensively" means nursing at least every four hours between daytime feedings and at least every six hours at night. Frequent nursing alters pituitary production of a couple of hormones that make you ovulate. We're not quite sure if pumping is as effective as nursing at the breast, so even if you are pumping frequently during the daytime, you may still get your period back.

The introduction of formula supplementation, the baby sleeping "through the night," or the introduction of solid foods spaces out the time between breastfeeding and can cause you to ovulate and get your period (and that means return of your fertility!).

So then, does the return of your period mean that your supply is bad or that you are going to have to wean? Nope. Sometimes there is a temporary drop in your supply, some nipple tenderness, and some kids don't like the taste of the milk during that time, but that's it. Nothing more serious going on.

CHAPTER 9.
MOTHER ISSUES — MILK SUPPLY

How Long Should I Nurse On Each Side?

Until the baby is done. It isn't the length of time, but the quality of the feeding that counts. My son and I both have a bowl of cereal every morning, the same amount, in the same size bowl. It takes him like 20 minutes to finish off the bowl, whereas I inhale it in about 45 seconds. It's the same bowl of cereal. My point: Time is not as helpful as it may seem.

There are many extraordinary things about breastmilk. Chief among them is that the composition of the milk changes from the first feeding in the morning to the last feeding at night and from the beginning of each feeding to the end.

At the start of each feeding, the first milk the baby gets is called the foremilk, which is designed to quench thirst. It is lower in calories and high in lactose. Lactose is a very important sugar that contributes to human brain development, helps absorb iron and calcium, and promotes the growth of a healthy gut.

At the end of each feeding, while the lactose concentration stays the same, the milk becomes higher in fat. This milk is called the hindmilk, and it is higher in calories because of its fat content. The more hindmilk the baby gets, the longer the baby should go between feedings. And nighttime feedings have more fat, promoting longer periods of sleep. You'll know when the baby gets the hindmilk—your child will come off the breast looking a little funny, totally zonked. I refer to it as the "milk buzz."

If we feed the baby, as many women were told "15 minutes on a side," we artificially limit the time the baby gets on the breast. Mom gets sore nipples because she has to break an often strong suck, and the baby gets lots of foremilk and not a lot of hindmilk. Too much foremilk gets the baby lots of lactose, to the point where there isn't enough of the enzyme to break it all down, and the baby starts to show signs of lactose overload, like gas and really frequent watery stools. Plus, since the foremilk is lower in calories, the baby is eating all the time. Inevitably, mom feels like her milk isn't "good enough" or she starts examining her diet for the cause of the gas.

All we have to do is let the baby decide when they are done. The baby should get soup, salad, meat, potatoes, and dessert on the first side, and an after dinner drink on the second, if he wants it. Just begin the next feeding on the opposite side. And if your baby likes to snack, then you could potentially assign them one breast for a three-hour period of time, so baby gets some hindmilk. Plus, until the baby is six weeks old or so, he will stop eating and start to go to sleep, not when he is full, but when the flow of milk slows down. So, to get the baby to eat longer on one side, you have to keep the milk flowing. You can do a technique called breast compression to help you out. It involves massaging the breast during the feeding, coaxing milk into the baby's mouth. A good squirt of breastmilk to the suck reflex on the baby's palate will get him to suck if he is still going to feed.

MY MILK SUPPLY IS LOW—WHAT CAN I DO? (OR AN APPROACH TO LOW MILK SUPPLY FROM PREGNANCY THROUGH THE FOURTH B)

When approached by a mom with a true low milk supply, I first want to consider what needs to happen in order for a woman's breasts to make milk. I've discussed this before, but it would be helpful to review the physiologic process here, before moving on to possible solutions to a true low milk supply. So let me examine the stages.

Pregnancy

So, first we need breasts that go through normal estrogen-mediated growth during puberty. Then we need the pregnant breast to create the ducts, lobules, and supporting structures to create milk. These are created by prolactin, progesterone, and chorionic gonadotropin (HCG—the thing that pregnancy tests check for). Breast growth in pregnancy, unlike puberty, has little to do with estrogen.

Estrogen in pregnancy helps increase prolactin, the hormone that makes milk. The creation of milk also needs insulin to help increase the number of supporting structures. Cortisol needs to be around to help with the formation of alveoli.

Breastmilk can be secreted by 16 weeks of gestation, but isn't because milk secretion is held in check by progesterone and lactogen, both of which are formed by the placenta. The receptors that help with making milk like both prolactin and placental lactogen, but usually the placental lactogen hogs most of them.

So far, we need adequate insulin and sensitivity to it, progesterone and lactogen (in other words, a working placenta), estrogen, prolactin, and cortisol. One of the questions we can ask when we approach low milk supply is "Did you experience breast growth during pregnancy?" If we get "no" as an answer, we have several culprits. Maybe the mother has hypoplastic (underdeveloped) breasts from puberty. Perhaps we are dealing with poorly controlled diabetes, which would affect insulin and its actions. Maybe we have a mother with polycystic ovarian syndrome (PCOS), where the body doesn't respond to insulin the way it's supposed to. And there are many hormones that control prolactin. An abnormality of any of them may impact supply. If the answer to our breast growth question is "no," then we might need to set some realistic expectations for milk supply. If we didn't create the structures, we'll have milk production issues.

Regulation

The hormones responsible for the regulation of milk creation are oxytocin and prolactin. Oxytocin is a product of the posterior (back part) pituitary gland. Prolactin comes from the anterior (front) part of the pituitary gland. Oxytocin can be released under a variety of circumstances and doesn't need direct suckling at the breast to work. It is responsible for the milk ejection reflex (the "let-down"). It can be inhibited by stress. Cool plan. If you were running away from tigers, you'd hardly want to be leaving a trail of milk behind you. They could track you.

Prolactin, however, is only released by stimulation of the breast. The fourth intercostal (literally "between ribs") nerve is responsible for taking the information about suckling to the brain. Prolactin is the only hormone that is constantly prevented from being released. Most hormones have a mechanism where if it gets too high, something lowers it. Or if it gets too low, something increases it. But not prolactin. Dopamine keeps it in check until suckling begins. The info from the nerve comes in, dopamine decreases, and prolactin does its stuff.

Prolactin can be affected by insulin, cortisol, thyroid hormones, parathyroid hormones, and growth hormone. So low milk supply issues here could come from insulin issues, again, or disorders of any of that list of hormones. I often check thyroid hormones in mothers who have supply issues I can't seem to get a handle on.

Low milk supply may also occur because of previous trauma (car accidents, biopsies...) or breast surgery that may impact the fourth intercostal nerve. Breast reduction comes into play here because when they do that surgery, they often remove the nipple entirely (sorry for the visual) and those nerves are cut. When that happens, the brain has a very, very hard time getting the suckling information from the breast and no prolactin would be released. Those nerves do grow back, slowly. (We estimate about 1mm per year.) If the mother has areolar sensation, we have a chance of achieving a milk supply, maybe not a full one (again, setting realistic expectations), but something.

Dopamine-enhancing medications, like many of the medications used to treat ADHD and the antidepressant/ smoking cessation medication Wellbutrin, may cause some decrease in supply because they increase dopamine and, therefore, may decrease prolactin.

And tigers. Define "tiger" however you'd like, but stress of any sort can inhibit the milk ejection reflex. Alcohol can inhibit oxytocin as well. Alcohol is another discussion, however, so just know for milk supply purposes that it can make it hard to express milk. I see that as a good plan actually.

The First Several Days After Childbirth

During pregnancy, the cells that make up the structure of the breast are leaky—things can pass between them. This also happens during episodes of mastitis and when you wean and the breast structures involute (go away), but that's for another day.

At birth, those cells get lots less leaky. The "gap junctions" close. This keeps sodium and chloride from getting in and lactose from getting out. Over the next couple of days, lactose, which is a sugar, pulls water in with it and the milk "comes in," which is a term, as I have mentioned, that I really don't like.

What makes this happen? The placenta comes out and with it progesterone levels drop way down. With progesterone gone, milk synthesis increases. Cool. Then we need insulin, prolactin, and cortisol to continue production. So the milk secretion in the first few days is an endocrine process; it is not "demand and supply" until the third or fourth day, when milk supply drops if the milk is not removed from the breast. The baby still needs to nurse frequently and with a correct latch, get skin-to-skin, and all those good things, but the process here is endocrine, so it's very, very unusual for a mother to have "nothing." Colostrum can be secreted without the baby's help.

Poor supply here? Well, it can be caused by things that keep progesterone around, like retained placental fragments. And here's where we would encourage women to be educated about Depo-provera as a contraceptive. Depo is a progesterone hormone, maybe not the exact hormone the placenta makes, but awfully close. We have no idea who will have a drop in supply because of that Depo injection. And as far as I know, we have no Depo-sucking machine that can get that three month injection out of your system if it does affect your supply. If you choose to use contraception right after birth, and that's up to you, we'd suggest that you try something like a progestin-only pill that you can stop if it drops your supply. Better yet, barrier methods might be better. (And kudos for wanting to have sex!)

Again, insulin is very necessary here. If the mother had insulin dependent or gestational diabetes or PCOS, we may see a delay in the transition to a larger milk supply. If she needed metformin or other medication to get and stay pregnant, I usually encourage mothers to stay on it.

C-sections (which I'd place in the category of stress) may cause a delay in transitioning to a larger milk supply. We're not sure what the mechanism is here, but I would guess that the mom's body is protecting her (she did just have abdominal surgery) before she tries to care for someone else. I think postpartum heavy bleeding falls into this section as well.

A Low Supply After the First Few Days

Now we have demand and supply. We need a good latch. And if we have a poor supply here, the first things on the list are latch, latch, latch, latch... you get the point. The more milk out, the more you get. Poor supply here can come from any number of latch issues and things like tongue-tie or other baby anatomical issues, like cleft lip and palate.

What's the biggest factor here other than latch for poor supply? Confidence.

We mess this up in every way we can. My three "B"s—birthweight, bilirubin and blood sugar—come into play. Maybe I need another "B"—bad advice. We get something called "insufficient milk supply syndrome" (which I'll discuss in more depth in the next section) in many women. And yes, I'm an allopathic doctor—we named a disease process after confidence-rotting interventions. This is where we need to support mom, give a consistent message, avoid supplementation, avoid solid foods until six months, and keep cheerleading, no matter who you are in relationship to that new mom.

'I THINK I'M NOT MAKING ENOUGH MILK' OR THE SYNDROME OF INSUFFICIENT MILK SUPPLY AND THE WISDOM OF YODA

Intentional title. I think it's really called "perceived insufficient milk supply," but I'm an allopathic doctor, and as I understand that description, I need a disease to talk about. I'm also a big geek, and as I understand that definition, I should be able to quote Star Wars. Hands down, my favorite quote is from Yoda in "The Empire Strikes Back" when Luke is training to be a Jedi in a swamp. Luke is having a hard time with this Jedi stuff. Yoda says, *"Do, or do not. There is no try."* Hearing it quoted by Shemar Moore on "Criminal Minds" didn't hurt to impress it upon my memory.

I went on and on about possible physiologic explanations for low milk supply a few pages ago, so this isn't written about those mothers who either have medical explanations for low supply or can't find an explanation for their actual low supply. It is for those mothers that *misperceive* their actual supply.

This idea that mothers are supplementing and weaning because they feel as if they have "no milk" or *"I can't satisfy him"* is as important as Star Wars. It's a cultural phenomenon. It's everywhere. It's marketed and grosses lots of money. And the story is passed down from generation to generation. And if you have no Yoda to inspire you, well, there may be a dark side. At about 3:00 am. When you don't understand what the baby is doing. And you are starting to believe all those subversive messages that are so pervasive.

According to Gatti (2008) about 35% of women cite perceived insufficient milk supply as a reason for weaning. Other authors go as high as 80 percent. The most common reason for the perception that a mother's body can't make enough milk for her baby is lack of confidence and this idea that she can't satisfy her baby. Crying is a big deal, too. And moms always seem to blame the crying on themselves first, without looking for other reasons the baby might cry—like an older sibling who just knocked them over.

So what else may lead to the "dark side" thoughts. Well, lack of social support for one. Interestingly, one study put the blame squarely on the mother-in-law's disapproval. Perhaps it's marketing practices of infant formula companies. Ya, I'm going to skip the "perhaps." Maybe it's hospital practices, like separation of the mother and infant, or poor, evidenceless – based practices. Or maybe providers get in the way with my "Three Bs" of bilirubin, birthweight and blood sugar. Maybe it's under-education of what a normal newborn is supposed to do. Of course, maybe "I don't have enough milk" is a socially acceptable way to stop breastfeeding.

What it is, at its root, is lack of confidence, for whatever reason. That the body that created the beautiful baby can't possibly satisfy him.

As wise as I believe Master Yoda is, I'm going to quote myself here (you'll recognize the quote, if you've read this far): Why don't we trust our bodies postpartum? I don't know. But I hear over and over that the formula is because "I am just not satisfying him." Of course you are. Babies don't need to "eat" all the time—they need to be with you all the time—that's the ultimate satisfaction.

Helping Your Supply

These are not tips for those of you trying to establish milk supply, unless you've talked about it with your healthcare provider first. I'm including this info up for moms trying to increase the amount they pump at work, or other scenarios where the supply had been OK, but now is dwindling.

Before we use these medications/supplements, we have to make sure the latch is OK, we're using breast compression, we've tried pumping after feedings to increase breast stimulation, and that there isn't some other reason the supply has dwindled, like increased stress (hah!), poor diet, lack of sleep (double HAH!), starting on an estrogen-containing birth control pill, thyroid problems, pregnancy, oversupply, pseudoephedrine cold medications (or any other medication for that matter). Actually, one of the bigger reasons to have your supply drop off is pregnancy. That's an easy test to check and a good place to start.

Usually, the supply is lower because you are sleeping longer at night and not getting as much stimulation at the breast or you're back at work and can't pump as much as you'd like. Fix that first. (A first sign that you aren't getting as much breast stimulation is getting your period back...frequent breast stimulation keeps the period away, but as soon as you consistently go longer than maybe four hours or so without feeding/pumping, your period may come back.)

Plus, you make a bunch more milk than you need in the early weeks, and then you start to drop off a little, dipping into the stored supply. Everybody gets nervous when that happens, but we expect that drop-off to occur. Doesn't mean we like it—I saw every frozen bag thawed as a sign of failure. Really—thank goodness I married a psychiatrist.

There is great info on all three of these meds on www.breastfeedingonline.com that I'm not going to repeat here. You should look it up.

And remember, that along with these, you need to eat protein, drink until your thirst is quenched (but not more than that—too much water decreases supply!), sleep (nothing fixes problems like a good nap), and give yourself a break. Keep in mind that a full 25% of the women in the U.S. never even try breastfeeding. It's the right thing to do and often the right thing to do is not easy.

Fenugreek: This is a non-prescription herbal supplement that increases milk supply by decreasing an inhibitor of prolactin, the hormone that makes milk. It sometimes makes you smell like maple syrup and can upset your stomach, but can really boost your supply. In fact, this stuff is good enough where we may not have to do anything else to increase your milk supply. The starting dosage is one or two 600-625 mg capsules every day for a few days. If you have no stomach upset, then bump up the dose to three capsules three to four times a day. Blessed thistle, another herbal supplement, can help with the stomach upset if it occurs. A recent review of these herbs by the Academy of Breastfeeding Medicine shows that they probably don't help. That's what makes all the other steps before this so important.

Domperidone: This one is a prescription medication in the United States. It works by increasing prolactin levels. There currently is a lot of confusion about this medication in the U.S., but it has been given "orphan drug" status, and that is going to help us do the studies needed to understand more about this drug and how it can help breastfeeding mothers. I personally feel it is a much safer alternative to Reglan (metaclopromide), which is sometimes offered as an alternative.

Reglan (metaclopromide): This one is (usually) covered by insurance, but I've had less luck with it. In fact, I'm not using it much, if at all, anymore. It's similar to Domperidone, in that it is a prescription GI drug that also increases milk supply, but it has some theoretical side effects that most of us find annoying: fatigue and depression. Those of you I've had on this medication had some modest improvement in your supply, but many of you were really tired. I'm not going to recommend a dose here, because in my experience, it has too many side effects to even recommend a dose.

WHY IS MY BREASTFED BABY SO CRANKY? (POTENTIAL EXPLANATION NUMBER ONE: OVERSUPPLY)

One of the under-recognized reasons for weaning is because a baby is getting too much milk. I think that it's a reason for weaning because moms go to their pediatricians (instead of to a lactation consultant) for the symptoms, and it gets diagnosed as reflux, or colic, or a sinus infection or something, and the kids wind up at allergists or GI docs who tell them to wean.

My colleagues and I have spent ages trying to come up with a way to describe this, so we can test our theories. One problem is that too much milk and an aggressive let-down reflex don't always happen together, but when this set of symptoms is described, they are often lumped together. Another is that each kid responds differently to too much milk. Some just aren't bothered by it, and some are—so much so that weaning is nearly inevitable.

So it's called "oversupply" or "hyperlactation" or "overactive milk ejection," and it can be a mixed blessing. You sure get to store up a bunch of milk if you are pumping, but if you don't remove the milk adequately, you can get recurrent plugged ducts and mastitis and other unpleasantness.

We don't know really why it happens (I have my theories though). The ability to produce breastmilk exists on a spectrum. On one end, we have moms who aren't able to produce enough milk. I can usually help with that, or at least attempt to explain it. On the opposite side of the spectrum are the moms who can't ever seem to be empty, leaking through clothes and bedding, pumping crazy amounts of milk, even when their obviously full baby is done eating. Maybe it's from too much pumping (one theory). Maybe it's because there is something really cool about those moms we haven't figured out yet. Some people say these women are "blessed." I bet the people who can still pump eight ounces after the baby eats aren't very comfortable, and probably don't feel so blessed.

Mothers who overproduce breastmilk can have plugged ducts, recurrent mastitis, and breast abscesses. Infants of mothers with an oversupply of breastmilk (or whatever we call it) will often choke and sputter at the breast, and pull off and reattach themselves to the breast as they attempt to control the flow of milk. This can happen even at the end of the feeding, since the milk ejection reflex ("let-down") occurs several times during a feeding. I've seen these kids actually use their hands to push away the breast. They sometimes bite to slow the flow and often get on the breast, suck a few times, and then cry. That may get diagnosed as reflux. They always sound "congested" because there is always food banging around the back of their nose. You can try to suck that noise out, but it's food, not snot.

These babies feed frequently, gain weight very quickly, are often "colicky," and have explosive watery bowel movements. Mothers of these children are often told to wean the baby since the child is "allergic" to the milk. Many kids wind up on antacids (for the reflux), are given all sorts of advice for "colic," and the moms wind up on diets of boiled chicken and rice because of food allergies. Some moms may have been treated for yeast. Many just wean. These babies can be managed without having to wean. Plus, breastmilk allergy is extremely rare if it even occurs. And yeast is not invasive. It stays on top of the skin.

Overabundance of maternal milk should be distinguished from other reasons for breast fullness, such as engorgement, which may be related to a poor latch and poor milk transfer from the breast. Usually, the baby is gaining like crazy when the mom has breast fullness from overproduction. Breast fullness from engorgement should be managed with the help of someone experienced in assessing breastfeeding complications.

Before we try to fix the problem, you could try positioning the baby more upright, facing the breast, so at least they won't get a big spray of forcefully released milk while they are lying on their back. I would suggest, if you can do it, latching the baby as you normally would and then reclining back, so you are almost laying down and the baby is coming at the breast from the top, taking away the effect of gravity. It takes some practice, but it really helps decrease the amount of air the baby is taking in, thereby decreasing the burping and gas stuff. And put your feet up. One of my theories has to do with blood pressure, and nursing with your feet up or while lying down on your side raises your blood pressure and may slow the squirting. (My theory. Lots of clinical experience; no data yet, so don't quote me, at least for this part.)

It's the aggressive milk ejection reflex that makes babies sputter. You would, too, if you got a big blast of something in the back of your throat. You might even make choking noises. You might throw up and perhaps burp loudly. This oversupply/aggressive milk ejection isn't any fun for the kids. Most breastfeed kids don't burp well or at all since they can control the rate of flow from the breast. These kids can't control the flow of milk, and they will burp with the best of 'em.

We can fix the oversupply, if you want to, with a little "lactoengineering." You only make as much milk as is removed—"demand and supply" rather than "supply and demand," so demand less. Feed several times on one side and let the other side stay more full. Make sure that you don't let the other breast get so full that it's going to explode since that's what causes the plugged ducts and mastitis. Pump it until you're comfortable, but not to empty. Pumping to empty makes you make more milk.

A couple of things happen when you use just one side. First, we work on foremilk/hindmilk imbalances. We're not really supposed to be using these terms anymore, but I think they are helpful.

Foremilk, as I have mentioned, is the thirst-quenching milk in your breast, ready to go at the beginning of the feeding. It has lots of lactose, but not much fat, so it's low in calories. Lactose is very important. It helps with the intestinal absorption of calcium and iron. It helps promote the growth of good bacteria in the gut. And probably most importantly, it is a sugar that attaches to a lipid needed for brain development.

Hindmilk, at the end of a feeding, is higher in calories because it's higher in fat. The amount of fat slowly increases over a feeding, releasing a gut hormone called cholecystokinin (CCK) that tells your brain you are full. If you don't get that fat, you don't get CCK, and you keep eating. If you do several feedings on one breast, then there is less foremilk to get through and the baby might just feel full. You'll know when the baby gets to the hindmilk because they come off the breast looking verrrrry satisfied. This process works on opioid receptors, you know, like morphine. That state of enough-fat contentment I call the "milk buzz." The baby who is blown off the breast by a squirt after a let-down is different than the one enjoying the milk buzz. The kids with the milk buzz are out, hard to arouse. Kids squirted off wake up right away, if they even slept. Those kids should go on the same breast until you see the buzz.

If mom has a lot of milk, the kid get lots of milk, and lots of lactose. Lactose is a sugar. Lots of sugar delivered to your stomach makes your stomach empty faster. Fat makes it empty slower. Lots of lactose leaves the stomach, heads to the intestine in a big blop, and just can't all be digested because it's moving fast and there may not be enough enzyme to break it all down. This is often mistaken for lactose intolerance, which is really, really, really rare in infancy. The kids then get gassy, have explosive poops, and get really irritable. Most moms blame something in their diet. It's probably that the baby doesn't know they are full. They gain weight like crazy and are always at the breast. We just need to make the baby know they are full.

I'm not a fan of nipple shields, but this may be one time where, if position changes don't help, that they may work. They might serve as a "breakwater" to slow things down a bit and make the feeding more pleasant. We can also use drugs, although this is a desperate measure. For example, while pseudoephedrine is compatible with breastfeeding, just one 60 mg capsule can suppress milk production. Estrogen-containing birth control pills may also help.

If this goes on without us realizing that the kids are getting blasted, they may start to refuse the breast. Wouldn't you? If you were getting squirted every time you ate something (even if it's something you really loved), wouldn't you try to avoid it? Maybe. Or the kids may "play" at the breast, latching on, pulling off, latching on, pulling off... you could get the idea that the child doesn't like your milk, or that you ate something bad, or that you don't have any or enough milk when your child is actually developing defensive maneuvers to protect themselves from the big squirt. They may bite to slow the flow and that might be an important cause of nipple pain.

Also, if this quick flow of milk heads through the gut, poorly digested, it's not much of a stretch to think the gut may not work perfectly and other intolerances may show up. I've seen cow milk protein become the most problematic, but other countless things could be blamed. Lactose feeds the good bacteria in the gut. If that sugar doesn't feed those good bacteria, they might not grow, may not digest things well, and cause the kids pain. Probiotics may be very helpful as we fix the flow.

And if you make it through all of those symptoms without weaning, your older baby may have learned some adaptive skills when it comes to eating and drinking. They may not like solid foods fed to them—they may want to control their intake themselves. I think I've seen plenty of kids with oral aversion symptoms because they learned to adapt to mom's really fast milk flow. Again, though, I've seen plenty of kids who just don't mind at all.

Of course, we don't necessarily have to fix the oversupply because not every kid is bugged by the fast flow. It may come in handy for later use, such as a return to the workplace. We can also consider donating extra milk to our local milk bank, in my case the Mother's Milk Association of Wisconsin in Madison. (You can search for yours online at www.HMBANA. org.)

CHAPTER 10.
MOTHER ISSUES — SORE NIPPLES

NIPPLE PAIN: WHY DOES THIS HURT SO MUCH?

Nipple pain is no small problem. Many new mothers describe the pain right from the first feeding. Many more experience it in the first week. And many don't seek help and wean. I hope that with constant, continual, annoying encouragement, you will seek help if you are one of those that has this pain. We know from research and from practical experience that proper positioning and an appropriate latch can save your nursing experience. Pain is a powerful motivator to quit, I get it. But there are those whose entire job it is to make your nursing experience a great experience, and they can help. And we know it makes a difference.

A good latch doesn't compress the nipple. If your baby comes off the breast and the nipple is compressed (like a new lipstick), then we know the tongue was in the wrong spot, touching the nipple and causing trauma. That trauma, if it continues, can lead to worsening sores and may be a jumping off point for infection.

Besides a poor latch and infection, what other things can cause pain? Well, the list is long. At about day four to six, the shape of the breast changes because the volume of milk within it gets larger, sometimes to the point where we would say the breast is "engorged." It's one thing for the tongue to get to the right position, under the nipple, and compress the milk ducts and extract milk. It's a totally different story all together if the baby is trying to suck on a basketball. That change in the contour of the breast with engorgement may make a good latch hard to achieve. Some women find that hand expression or pumping a little milk from the breast can make it more compressible, allow the baby to latch more easily, and reduce the nipple trauma and pain.

What if the baby's tongue can't get to the right spot because it has limitations in how far it can elevate, move side to side, or extend. That's called *ankyloglossia* or "tongue-tie," and occurs when a small flap of skin connects the base of the tongue to the floor of the mouth. Again, we need someone who can assess that on your baby to see if it might be the problem causing the pain, so you have to ask for help (annoying yet?), but it's relatively easy to fix in the right hands and can make a world of difference.

Older babies may have developed some adaptations to their latch over time. This especially happens when the milk flow is really fast. If you were gulping instead of sipping your drink, after a while you might do something to make the experience more pleasant. For a baby struggling with a fast milk flow, biting the nipple and pulling back on it is one way to slow down the flow. This can lead to trauma and pain—pain that may not have been there when your supply wasn't as large when your nursing relationship started. Regulation of an "oversupply" of milk or an aggressive let-down can help the baby stop using those protective maneuvers, and stop the trauma and subsequent pain.

Pain can also be caused by underlying conditions that have nothing to do with the latch or the baby. For example, mothers with a condition called "Reynaud's phenomenon" can experience it on their nipples as well. Reynaud's phenomenon happens when a finger, toe, or in our case, nipple is exposed to cold. A characteristic color change sequence happens. The nipple (for our purposes) turns white (from lack of blood flow due to blood vessel constriction), then blue (from oxygen deprivation while the blood vessel is constricted), and then red (when the blood vessel opens again and the area flushes with blood.) This type of nipple pain is treated as Reynaud's phenomenon is typically treated—trying to avoid unnecessary exposure to cold, using fish oils, or potentially using medications that dilate blood vessels.

Other conditions mothers can have that cause nipple pain are things like eczema, psoriasis, trauma from incorrect pump settings, and other stuff you'd just never think of in warmer places of the world, like frostbite.

So what do we know about nipple pain? Well, pain is not normal, so something is wrong. The first ten reasons on the list of why nipples might be sore is a poor latch. And as I may have said a million times before, the latch should not be painful, so finding a resource who is specifically knowledgeable about assessing a latch is really, really important.

If it's not the latch, and we're sure it's not the latch, then what else could it be? Potentially, the nipple tissue could be infected. The culprit infectious agents are *staphylococcus aureus* (staph) or *candida albicans* (yeast). Both of these are found on your body normally. They don't usually cause infection unless there's a break in the integrity of the skin. The skin gets damaged, and these normally pretty harmless organisms can jump on, cause infection, and create pain. But, and here's the rub, how did the skin of the nipple get damaged? We need to go back to the latch again and make sure no trauma is occurring because of it, not only because a bad latch causes pain, but because the infections that can arise from a bad latch are also painful. Pain is a tiger.

The organism most likely to cause infection is *staph*. We seem to blame yeast more, though. More on this next.

The Trouble With Yeast. Too Much Diagnosis. Too Little Data.

Nipple pain is caused by two major things: a poor latch and a bacteria called *staph aureus*. Other things can cause pain: vasospasm (or a constriction of the blood vessels of the nipple), Reynaud's phenomenon (where the nipple turns white, red, then blue), pump trauma, certain skin conditions, tongue-tie, pregnancy, and other infections, like yeast. It's not meant to be an all-inclusive list, but you get the idea. Lots of things cause pain.

But we do know from lots of studies that the vast majority of pain is due to a poor latch (and probably vasospasm after the latch is fixed) and *staph aureus*. And the *staph* can't get there unless the skin is broken, and the skin gets broken from nipple injury, so back to the latch. The point is bacteria are much more common as a cause of nipple pain, but we blame yeast for everything.

So, a little on yeast. The typical symptoms described for yeast are redness, itching and burning of the nipples, and shooting pain in the breast. The diagnosis is often made by looking at the nipple and correlating it with symptoms. No culture is done, and if it was, it's probably useless. Lactoferrin in human milk makes culturing yeast from milk very difficult unless the right technique is used. And you have to culture nipples very carefully and interpret the results carefully. Many studies have shown that women with no nipple pain will often grow yeast on a skin culture. It also doesn't "invade" tissues; in normal people, it stays on the surface of tissues. That's why the diagnosis of "ductal yeast" has never made sense to me. The yeast would have to invade to cause that pain. Dr. Hale's excellent study calls into very serious question whether ductal yeast exists (http://www.ncbi.nlm.nih.gov/pubmed/19500049).

Yeast is found naturally in everyone's GI tract, and it helps with the health of the GI tract. If you culture random people, you can get Candida (which I'm going to continue to call yeast) from the mouths of 31-55 percent of them. Yeast is everywhere. It only becomes a disease-causing agent when something else is wrong. For example, you got antibiotics and killed the good bacteria in your gut. Then the yeast overgrow and have a party. Or you have AIDS, are receiving chemo, or have otherwise really, really messed up your immune system.

In terms of treatment, there are no ("gold-standard") randomized controlled trials. Fluconazole (Diflucan) is often used. It can cause blood vessel constriction and make vasospasm symptoms worse. Expert opinion says treat mom and baby, even if one has no symptoms, but again, no data supports that practice. Sounds messy to me and maybe we should know we are treating yeast before we actually treat it. Because if we treat yeast and it isn't yeast, we are keeping that mother in pain unnecessarily. And pain causes weaning. We need to get this right for the sake of the dyad.

I haven't treated yeast for nipple pain in ages in my own practice because I know (and hopefully you do, too, now) that the overwhelming causes of nipple pain are related to poor latch and *staph*. I use Muciprocin (Bactroban) for the *staph* and fix the latch. But the women I care for who come to see me talk of "resistant yeast" and have been on numerous courses of yeast-treating things with no relief. How many times do we need to treat the same thing before we begin to think we have the wrong diagnosis?

In my practice, these symptoms are often oversupply, where the baby bites and pulls back, injuring the nipple. Some are missed significant tongue-tie. I've diagnosed more than a few women with Reynaud's phenomenon. I've seen pump trauma, usually from incorrect use (too high suction) or an old motor (too low suction), that resolves with a new or no pump. I've found a few pregnancies (much to the surprise of the mom...eek). One mother was pumping in her car in January, and I'm pretty sure her "yeast" was frostbite.

I'm not saying nipple yeast doesn't exist. But it shouldn't be our first or even our second guess.

Nipple Shields: Life Saver, Supply Wrecker, or Just Another Tool for Nursing Mothers?

I confess, I didn't know what a nipple shield was back in the day when I was still a very smart, but breastfeeding "knowledge-challenged" pediatrician. I did know that whatever they were, they were bad. Very bad. "Never" use them under any circumstances. Ever.

Later when my niece was born in a hospital hundreds, nay thousands, or millions of miles away from me, imagine my horror as I found out that she needed a nipple shield to latch. This was bad. I didn't know why, but it had to stop. So, as unsupportively as I could imagine (in retrospect), I told my sister to stop using that thing! I hadn't met my niece yet, but I knew that she was less than five pounds soaking wet and that nipple thingy was going to ruin her chances of getting into the Ivy League.

One of my dearest friends in the world needed to use a shield when her second child was born. She asked for one when her third was born and was told "no" by the staff caring for her in the hospital. To me, it just was further proof that their use was fraught with problems.

I'm smarter now, at least I'm less breastfeeding-challenged, and I know better than to use the words "never" or "always" and to deny a request without providing education and informed consent. And I've heard too many stories of success to discount the benefits of nipple shields for some mothers and babies. But the fact remains that we have no guidelines for nipple shield use. We have few studies rigorously done that show they are effective.

A nipple shield is a gadget that is placed over the nipple and areola area. It looks like a nipple (sort of) or a sombrero, but it is made of plastic, and there are different types. You can get them online and over-the-counter. The problem with them stems from studies (with flaws in the method in which they were done) that concluded the use of the shield could decrease milk supply, were associated with more supplementation, and led to early weaning.

That meant that if they were to be used, the dyad using them would need to be carefully followed, but many mothers were getting them and no follow up was scheduled. I'm not sure the logical result of that should be a compete ban on their use, but, well, they were highly discouraged. Of course, those studies were with older versions of the shield, and other research (with flaws in the method in which they were done) with newer versions of the shield suggested this wasn't as a big a problem as we thought. But many of those same concerns exist. We honestly don't know the short-term or long-term effects of nipple shield use.

Nipple shields are often given out in the nursery for "flat" nipples. My guess (no data, so definitely flawed study method) is that the nipples are puffy. And if that's the case, this might be something to try.

They are often given out for a poor latch as a quick fix to a more complex problem, but we need to remember basics: skin-to-skin, baby-led latch, biological nurturing, and asking for help from someone who is board certified in lactation, an "IBCLC." The shield should not be a first step.

If it's given to you because your nipples are sore, then in addition to the shield, we need somebody to fix the underlying problem and be your cheerleader as you heal and transition back to the breast. (Find a Lactation Consultant!)

So, suggestions: If you are given a nipple shield, ask why. Informed consent for any intervention means that you are given the required information in an understandable manner that allows your voluntary participation and helps in making a decision for a course of action. Questions you can ask to help fulfill informed consent: *Why am I getting this thing? How long do I use it? How will it help? Might it hurt? What other things might I try? What type of follow up do I need?*

If you are given a shield and it works, well, cool. You need follow up by somebody who knows something about breastfeeding, so we can work on the underlying issue that initially caused the need for the shield.

If you were given a shield and don't like it, well, let's get you some assistance and fix whatever the issue is that requires a gadget to fix it, so you can go gadget-less.

Shields are meant to be temporary solutions. If you are still using it when your baby is months old, we really should be able to help you stop using it, if you want us to.

If you are given a shield, it works well, your baby is growing and you're happy, but everyone around you is like "ooooooh, those things are bad," you have my permission to hear everything that person says after that in the voice of Charlie Brown's teacher. (Do you remember that voice, or am I showing my age?)

CHAPTER 11.
MOTHER ISSUES — RETURNING TO WORK

I'M GOING BACK TO WORK. HOW CAN I GET READY TO PUMP?

When I went back after having my oldest, I cried every day for about seven weeks, and I never even tried to pump. With my next two, I was ready, and even though it wasn't the easiest thing in the world, I pumped. I hope to get you ready to go back—to life, to work, and to your daily routine, if that's possible, and I'm going to include some of the experiences other moms in my practice have had.

Before the Baby Comes

I think it makes sense to talk to your employer and find out what opportunities you'll have to pump. If there is a lactation program at your company, then get the details. If there isn't, ask.

Here's some advice from women who've been in your shoes and how things worked out for them.

From Tori: *I presented the problem to the HR manager—a man, talk about uncomfortable. Basically, I told him that we weren't expected to prepare our OWN lunches in the bathroom—why should I be expected to prepare my son's meals in the bathroom? This was a company where even the president was in a door-less cubicle, and there were only two offices that had real walls and locks on the doors, and they were both in HR. The response really surprised me. I could not believe how accommodating they were. They put locks on the doors and blinds in the windows of two conference rooms. The HR manager also said that if both of those conference rooms were being used during my breaks, I could use his office. I don't work there anymore, but to my knowledge, those rooms are still being used by nursing moms. And all I had to do was ask. I couldn't believe the ladies before me resorted to the bathroom. If they would have just asked, those rooms could have been setup that way so much sooner.*

If other women at your company have been able to successfully pump, ask them where they pumped, where they cleaned the parts. You'll need to know if there is a refrigerator to store your milk or if you need to bring a cooler. Find out if your employer has flex-time, part time, or at home working options, since the less pumping you have to do, the happier your work experience will be.

After the Baby, Before Going to Work

I have lots of people, right in the nursery, ask me when they can start to pump to store milk for when they go back to work. And I know how much anxiety is caused when you don't have enough "milkcicles" stored up. But, at least in the first couple of weeks after the baby comes, your "job" is to get to know your baby. Forget about the pump and let the baby do the work of getting your supply up. The kids have a little software program in their heads that tells them to eat a lot, even when they are not hungry, in those first couple of weeks. If we mess up that program, we can wind up with a milk supply that does not meet the baby's needs...including the potential for too much milk. Too much milk can lead to the baby getting too much foremilk and not enough hindmilk, and becoming a gassy, cranky baby.

So priority one is establishing a good milk supply. This means the baby eats on demand for as long as they want and we avoid pacifiers and bottles until they are about three to four weeks of age.

If you give a bottle, I have no recommendation as to which one to use. Many kids won't take bottles. They will if they need to. We might need somebody else to give the bottle, because if the baby knows mom is around, they may not take the bottle. When they are near mom, they know what they want, and it isn't a hard piece of cold plastic. The baby's expectations for somebody who isn't mom are very different, and we have a bunch more success getting the kid to take the bottle when mom isn't the one giving it.

When you are an expert on breastfeeding (the baby is gaining weight and you two feel as if you have it down), then you can start saving milk for work. After each feeding, pump for about 10 minutes afterward. You won't get much at first, but the increased demand will create an increased supply over time. Then store what you pumped.

When you are looking for childcare providers, this is a good time to confirm that they will be comfortable giving your expressed milk.

Try to arrange going back to work on a Thursday or Friday, so you can do a short week and have a few trial runs.

Going Back After Maternity Leave

This is all about relaxing. Most likely, you're going to be pumping, unless you are lucky enough to have your baby visit you at the workplace. Pumped milk volume (actually all milk volume, but it's easier to notice when you are pumping) is greater when you are well rested and relaxed. And creating a relaxed setting at work is really important. I shopped online for jewelry when I was pumping. Here are some other ideas. (I like Lisa's advice about listening to me!)

From Lisa:

- *Do not look at the pump, do not watch the process, pay no attention to your breasts or what is happening down there! (Sounds funny, but it was a great help to me! This advice came from Dr. Jenny. Listen to her!)*

- *Have a picture of your little one. This relaxed me and helped with let down. Even just thinking about him/her can help.*

- *Read, surf the net, knit, scrapbook, etc. I found that if I really immersed myself into reading a book/magazine, it helped me relax and took my mind off what I was doing. In fact, sometimes I would be so engrossed I wouldn't even notice that I had pumped myself dry!*

From Tori:

We had two scheduled 15-minute breaks and a 30-minute lunch, so that's when I pumped. And to relax, I'd usually try to doze off during those times. The bells at the end of the breaks would always wake me back up again. They had a little kitchenette with a full size fridge, microwave, and sink available for employee use. I'd put the milk bottles in a brown paper lunchbag and put them in the fridge, and then rinse out the pump parts in the sink before I put them back in the bag for the next break. I washed the pump parts at home in the dishwasher every night.

From Mary:

The hardest part was relaxing and staying motivated to deal with that contraption everyday. I mostly went on the computer during those times to try to get my mind off of it. I would constantly worry about not getting enough milk...even though I never ran out. To stay motivated, I would just think about my son and the benefits it gave him...then there wasn't a question as to why I was doing all of this.

It's often easiest to nurse right before you leave for work and as soon as you get home. Make sure you tell your childcare provider to hold off on late afternoon feedings until you know when you can get home. It's a bummer when you come home and the baby has just eaten, because then you have to pump again, and feeding the baby at the breast is sooo much nicer. Or nurse at the daycare provider when you drop off and pick up. It's a great way to spend a little extra time with those who care for your child during the day.

Try to pump about every three or four hours when you are at work. But really, you don't need to find huge segments of time or uninterrupted time. Pumping twice or more in a row, 10 minutes to 30 minutes apart can work, too, and those interrupted clusters together would work as ONE pumping. You do what you can.

In general, you should expect to pump one ounce for every hour since you last fed or pumped, and that's a two-breast total. So if it's been three hours since you last pumped, then your next pumping should yield three ounces total. That's a general idea. I get worried when I say stuff like this because the general guideline may be taken as gospel. I'm giving you an idea, not a rule.

You should expect that the baby might take, at any one feeding, about half of what they weigh...meaning, if they weigh eight pounds, they'll take about four ounces. And maybe that's even inaccurate—they'll puke if they get more than they need. They certainly don't have to take that amount at any feeding. Again, this is a general guideline—an idea—not a rule.

Some kids do something called "reverse cycle nursing," where they eat more when they know you are going to be home and eat just enough to tide them over when you are at work. Your babysitter may tell you that your baby barely ate anything, and then the baby eats all the time when you are together. Smart kid.

THE RULES OF PUMPING

1. You can't look at the pump. Stress effects your let-down reflex (let's call it a milk ejection reflex—who wants to be let down???). If you are looking at the pump and thinking, "There's nothing coming out!" then your body says stress and your breasts don't work as well. (I found that shopping online for jewelry helped me relax when I was pumping. Other people read magazines, look at pictures of their kids...see the page on going back to work...)

2. You can't assume that what you get pumping is what the baby gets when you nurse. No breast pump mimics a baby's suck, and it's really hard to bond with a pump. Both factors combine to make your expressed milk less than what your baby can get. So, if you are pumping four ounces, your baby gets at least four ounces when they eat at the breast.

3. You cannot assume that your baby has been starved all along when they slam the bottle of expressed milk. Babies respond to a hard nipple with milk coming out, and that's what a bottle nipple is. The catch is that they cannot control the rate of flow like they can when they are nursing at the breast, so they eat very fast, whether they want to or not. This inability to regulate the flow of milk from a bottle leads to kids eating lots of air and was the reason we started burping our babies. Breastfed kids fed at the breast usually don't need to be burped.

4. You should be pumping as often as you can. Every three hours is optimal, but sometimes not do-able. Plus, clock watching causes stress, and stress is no good for anybody. Your pumping session should

be for what feels like 10 minutes and can be interrupted. It doesn't have to be 10 minutes, or 10 minutes straight. You can pump for what feels like five minutes, answer the phone, go to the bathroom, and pick up a little later and finish that pumping session.

5. You should pump one ounce for every hour since you last fed or pumped, and that's a two-breast total. So if it's been three hours since you last pumped, then your next pumping should (probably, maybe) yield three ounces total.

CHAPTER 12.
BABY ISSUES — POOP

Is My Breastfed Baby Constipated? (Or the Scoop on Poop, Part 1, for the Breastfed Newborn)

We have to start with a definition first. Constipation is passing stool that is as hard as rocks. It has nothing to do with the number of days kids go in between stools or the effort involved in passing the stool. What we do about it varies, depending on age and diet. Here, of course, we are looking specifically at breastfed infants in the first week of life.

Exclusively breastfed babies in the first few days of life should clear all the meconium stool by day of life four to five.

The stool transitions from black meconium to green, tarry meconium to brown to yellow. And if all is going well, the baby should be passing yellow stool on day four to five of life. The first milk the breasts make, colostrum, is a great laxative. The more colostrum the baby gets, the more poop they pass. **That means that any breastfed baby who does not stool (in the first week of life) is not getting enough milk.** This is an emergency, and your pediatrician would really like to hear from you and maybe see you and your baby.

Scoop On Poop, Part 2: What About Breastfed Infants After the First Week of Life?

Exclusively breastfed infants stool a bunch in the first few weeks of life, sometimes with every feeding. The stool can be quite watery and yellow or green.

Most (but not all) babies will have a change in the stool pattern after the first few weeks, sometimes abruptly. A likely reason that the stool output decreases later in lactation is that high oligosaccharide concentration of the first weeks, starts to drop off. I don't know if it's the only reason, but oligosaccharides are a main source of non-soluble fiber and therefore help in all that stool output in the first weeks. The concnetration of oligosacchirdes falls off after the first few months and may lead to a decrease in stool frequency. Nothing may change. Another pattern for breastfed infants in their second month of life is one "honey-fill-the-tub up-the-back-in-the-hair throw-away-that-outfit" stool a week.

Breastfeeding babies who are nursing well, gaining weight, and having at least six wet diapers a day are rarely truly constipated. No matter how much grunting or groaning they do or how much gas they pass.

Can I Use Gas Drops?

Sure, but let's make sure that it isn't an easy problem to fix. I don't recommend any particular brand. And remember, gas is normal. It's a sign that the gut is working properly. We all pass gas (put your hand on the bottom of your spouse all day and see what happens)! And how it smells tells me nothing. Gas is not usually fragrant at any age, so if your child passes "adult-smelling" gas, well, there you go.

If you are nursing, the most common problem causing an irritable, gassy, hungry baby is an imbalance of foremilk and hindmilk. And fixing it shouldn't be too hard. And don't go giving up chocolate or spicy foods or something without reading the question above. Most breastfed babies don't burp well, since they can't control the flow of milk well. Also, if you have a gassy, burping breastfed baby, maybe you have too much milk. Help for that is given earlier in this section.

CHAPTER 13.
BABY ISSUES — SLEEPY BABY

My Baby Keeps Falling Asleep at the Breast—What Can I Do?

Babies fall asleep at the breast all the time, and who can blame them? It's cozy, safe, and involves warm milk.

It's a problem, though, when mom wants to get up, put the baby down, and do something like shower or pee, and the baby wakes up and wants to eat again.

So what's up?

In the first 24 hours of life, newborns fall asleep because most got shoved though a very small hole and probably don't feel all that hot because of it. Plus, as medical professionals, we give many drugs to moms and babies that make both sleepy afterwards. There are very many reasons that I harp about babies going to breast as soon as possible after delivery; one of them is that newborns have about two hours of really awake time after delivery, and then sleep, soundly, for about the next 20 hours. Nursing during that 20 hours of sound sleeping can be very discouraging sometimes.

Why are we waking them up to begin with? In the first couple of weeks of nursing, mom needs to establish her milk supply. Suckling at the breast causes a release of the hormone prolactin, a necessary hormone for making milk. Prolactin levels rise during the first two weeks, eventually coming to a plateau after that. So frequent and effective sucking on the breast during that two weeks is important to establish an adequate level of prolactin. Prolactin starts to dip after three to four hours without stimulation at the breast, and that can make mom's milk supply less than necessary.

Infants in the first few weeks of life fall asleep because sometimes because mom is warm and snuggly, sometimes because they wanted to get back to mom is they were alone or held by someone else, or because the flow of milk slowed down or there is a true issue with milk supply. The idea, then, is to keep the flow of milk going. One technique to keep the milk coming is called breast compression and basically involves squirting the roof of the child's mouth with milk to keep him sucking.

As he nurses longer from one side, the composition of the mature milk (not colostrum) changes from low calorie to high calorie, low fat to high fat. The more high fat containing milk (hindmilk) he gets, the longer he theoretically will go in between feedings. This increase in hindmilk can help with gassiness and weight gain.

Another technique that works quite well, but one we wouldn't use for more than the baby's first few days of life, is called switch nursing, where you keep switching the baby back and forth between breasts during the same feeding. As the flow of milk slows and the baby's sucking subsequently slows, you switch to the other side. That way, we keep the flow of milk going during the feeding. Eventually, however, when your mature milk supply is established, this technique can lead to a foremilk/hindmilk imbalance, which leads to a gassy, hungry baby. Again, it's not a technique that we would do for much longer than the first week of life.

Other things to do:

- No feeding in a rocking chair as you'll both be asleep!

- Loosen or remove clothes and blankets.

- Change the baby's diaper.

- Learn to recognize the difference between light and deep sleep. Try not to awaken a baby in a deep sleep, but go for it when he is in a light sleep.

- Stimulate the baby's rooting reflex by stroking his cheek.

- Stroke under her chin from front to back.

Why Do Babies Wake Up So Much During the Night, Anyway?

Let's start with some biology. Nobody really understands why we sleep. What is pretty clear, though, is that something really important must be going on during sleep because we all do it, we all function poorly if we don't get enough, and the process has been preserved in humans for a really long time. Even when we were sleeping in caves and surrounded by tigers, sleeping was important enough to continue to do. And little kids spend most of their days sleeping.

Normal Sleep

To understand why sleep problems show up, we need to understand normal sleep. Probably the two most important stages of sleep are stage four sleep and REM (rapid eye movement) sleep.

In stage four sleep, you are completely unresponsive, with a disconnection between sensory information coming in and your ability to receive it. You can't hear people talking to you, you don't know your bladder is full, you don't smell smoke, and you can't tell if tigers are around. This is the prevalent sleep stage of the first part of the night, and the more tired you are, the longer you spend in stage four sleep. You have a really hard time being awakened or awakening from stage four sleep. Kids with disorders of stage four sleep will have sleepwalking, sometimes bedwetting, or night terrors.

In REM sleep, you have a complete loss of muscle tone. That's a good thing since you dream in REM sleep, and if you acted out your dreams, you could really hurt somebody or yourself. REM sleep happens towards the last part of the night. You can wake up easily from REM sleep. Kids with disorders of REM sleep have nightmares.

The stages of sleep, and there are more than just stage four and REM, are things we go through each night, but we go through them in cycles. Every 90 minutes or so, we actually wake up, check out our surroundings, and go back to sleep if everything feels safe.

So, as sleep has developed, one of the major issues surrounding it is safety. We could comfortably enter stage four sleep because other people were around us to keep us safe, and at least one person was probably in lighter stages of sleeping, so they could warn us if tigers were around. That sense of connection is really important to us now, even though we aren't really worried about predators. Disconnection from your sense of safety interferes with sleep.

Awakening about five to eight times a night is normal. We don't remember it, but we adjust our pillow and covers.

Kids develop sleep habits over time as they develop. Infants sleep about 20 hours a day. They frequently are awake at night, much as they were when they were in the womb. Just because we changed their scenery doesn't mean they know day from night. They can snuggle with us and sleep in our arms, and we aren't setting them up for anything bad.

We can't spoil kids in this age group, and I highly recommend holding and snuggling as much as possible. :) They should sleep on their backs, not on their sides or belly. The hormones that regulate the day night cycle kick in at about six to eight weeks of age. When they are about three to four months old, they have a decrease in night waking. That decrease is a brain development phenomenon and has nothing to do with solid foods, rice cereal, or quality of breastmilk.

But at five to nine months of age, there is an increase in night waking again. Many kids need their parents to feel safe because the brain pathways that sense strangers and fear are kicking in. The whole idea of kids sleeping in their own room, in their own bed, is a 20th century, pretty much American idea. You see, most species, since they all sleep, sleep in groups, with each member of the group in different stages of sleep, so predators don't sneak up on them without somebody knowing about it. And in many parts of the world, families sleep together, and the kids are never by themselves.

So...that's normal sleep. It's why babies wake up so much during the night...normal sleep, how we evolved, how our bodies are wired to work. Normal.

CHAPTER 14.
BABY ISSUES — GROWTH

Why Is My Breastfed Baby Getting Smaller on the Growth Charts?

When you come in for well visits, we weigh and measure your baby, and then plot them on a growth chart. We follow those percentiles over time to gauge how well your baby is growing and to see if we need to intervene if the baby isn't growing the way they used to.

The CDC growth curves, the one used most often in American offices, are based on population samples of the U.S. The information for the growth charts was collected from five separate surveys of the population of the U.S. done between 1963 and 1994. That data and the resulting growth curves show how kids *are* growing in the U.S. They are a growth reference.

Incidentally, the birth data comes from the two states that recorded birthweights on the birth certificate: Wisconsin (yeah!) and Missouri. The next set of data points come from information collected on two-month-olds. The growth chart lines between birth and two months aren't based on kids—they are a mathematically extrapolated part of the curve. There is some dispute about plotting the kids during weekly weight checks since the lines aren't based on any real kids.

The World Health Organization created a new set of growth curves to represent how kids *should* be growing. These curves are growth standards (that's not the same as a reference). They are often referred to as "the curve for a breastfed baby," but they aren't just curves for breastfed kids—they are based on how *all kids* should be growing.

The data for these standards were based on data collected on children from Brazil, Ghana, India, Norway, Oman, and the U.S. from 1997-2003. They were based on children receiving the best nutrition, without an environmental smoke exposure, and are meant to represent the best physiological growth in infancy and childhood. Breastfed infants do not "drop off" these curves.

Breastfed infants who drop percentiles are doing what they are supposed to do on the CDC curves. As time goes on during the first year of life, fewer and fewer children are being breastfed. We're trying to change that, but by nine months, very few children are still getting breastmilk, and when breastfed kids are compared to formula-fed ones, they will be smaller, leaner. Comparison of the CDC versus the WHO curves show that the differences in the "percentage" for breastfed kids starts as early as two months. Breastfed children will be "dropping off" of the CDC curve simply because they aren't being compared to a jury of their peers, so to speak. We have done a few consults for failure to thrive that have been fixed just by using the WHO curves instead of the CDC ones.

Breastfed kids in the U.S. almost always start dropping percentiles as they get older. And that can be alarming if you don't know why that's happening. This faltering on the growth curve can lead a mother to think her milk isn't "rich" enough or a physician to diagnose failure to thrive. If the baby was faltering because of the milk, though, why wouldn't that same child consume more complementary food to make up for lost calories? Maybe we aren't measuring the child on the right curve.

Fortunately, the CDC has now endorsed the use of the WHO curves for children from birth to two years of age. And they have lots of good info as to why they endorsed a product they didn't design.

For example:

- The WHO standards establish growth of the breastfed infant as the norm for growth.

- The WHO standards provide a better description of physiological growth in infancy.

(http://www.cdc.gov/growthcharts/who_charts.htm)

CHAPTER 15.
BABY ISSUES — INTRODUCING OTHER FOODS

Can I Give My Baby Juice?

The AAP feels pretty strongly about juice, and not much of it is a strong good feeling. The "Committee on the Use and Misuse of Fruit Juice in Pediatrics" (which sounds to me like something out of Harry Potter's Ministry of Magic!) has stated that juice is overused and can cause potential bad things. But I'll tell you, heading to the baby aisle at my local grocery store is quite an eye-opener. There is soooo much juice there that you have to figure kids need the stuff, right?

Well, maybe. If you've read this far and gotten to know me this well, you know I'm not going to be a juice cheerleader.

But in defense of juice:

- Juices that have ascorbic acid in them (you have to read the ingredients) can help with iron absorption if you drink them when you are eating food with iron in it.

- The vitamin C in fruit juice can help prevent cancer and heart disease.

- It can help fix constipation because it causes diarrhea.

Fruit juice is not the same as a fruit drink—fruit juices are better for you than fruit drinks, which are not good for you at all.

All the other stuff:

Juice started before six months of age is not necessary and can interfere with a child's hunger for food with real nutrition. If you are breastfeeding, there is nothing the baby needs besides breastmilk.

And kids older than six months of age still don't need juice. It can mess up their new incoming teeth, can replace good foods with nutrition in them, and cause diarrhea.

If you decide to give juice, use it as a way to get kids off the bottle. Put it in a cup. And as a practical tip, don't put it in a spill-proof cup—those were invented for us, not our kids. If you are a kid and have never used a cup, the mechanism you need to get stuff out of a spill-proof cup is going to be too hard to figure out. Let it spill on them, so they figure out how the thing works. Then go to the spill proof. Come to think of it, since I am advocating making a mess, use water, not juice.

If you give juice, don't give more than four to six ounces a day. And make it part of a snack, not something the kids get to walk around with all day.

They don't eat a whole lot of calories every day. They are really, really good (if they are left alone to regulate their intake) at taking in enough calories to grow. If a bunch of those calories come from juice, we have not done them any nutritional favors.

If you are giving juice for the vitamin C, give mashed or pureed fruit. Real fruit.

If you are going to give juice:

- Make it 100% fruit juice.

- Make sure the kids are older than six months.

- Give no more than four to six ounces a day (you can dilute that to six gallons if you want—just no more than four to six ounces of 100% stuff).

- Use a cup, not a bottle.

- Make sure it's fruit juice and not a fruit drink.

Is It Time to Feed My Baby Solid Food Yet?

The answer is it depends. But if your child is **four months to six months old,** sorry, still no solids. I know, everyone is pressuring you to start and that can be frustrating and annoying if we don't explain why we would prefer for you to wait. The American Academy of Pediatrics, the World Health Organization, and almost every other group concerned about the health and well-being of infants has said that six months is the recommended time for starting solid foods. Six months. There should be NO RUSH to start solids. The timing of this recommendation has nothing to do with developmental milestones. This is a recommendation based on good studies which tell us that waiting until six months can prevent chronic disease in the long-term.

If you have made the commitment to breastfeed, the AAP (of which I am a member) says that exclusive breastfeeding for the first six months of life is beneficial and desirable. Again, this is for long-term disease prevention for conditions like diabetes, but it also provides better infectious disease protection to your breastfed infant. Complementary foods are not necessary and may detract from the nutritional and infection-fighting benefits of breastmilk.

Now, the reality is that most breastfed kids have a "growth spurt" at about this time, and start getting up in the night (if they hadn't before). Breastmilk is supply and demand, and the kids are "demanding" to increase mom's supply. It does not mean the kids need solids. Solids don't make kids sleep. There is no sedative effect of rice cereal (since when did starch make a child sleep?), carrots, or peas.

And we should NOT be making decisions about solids based on sleep schedules. Four-month-olds may wake up and not be able to go back to sleep because they realize that there is a world out there. It is about safety, not hunger. We wake up and we are hungry, but we don't wake up because we are hungry.

I also know that four-month-olds are eating more and may not seem "satisfied" with what we just fed them. If they need more food, then it should be breastmilk. Giving cereal, or whatever, doesn't give them the nutrition they need at this age.

A child who is ready for solids should be trying to eat what's on your plate. Not just watching, but trying to get it. And that's rarely occurring before five months. The decision to start solids should have nothing, nothing, to do with sleep patterns. Nothing!

So when we decide the kids are ready for food, what food do we start with? The American tradition has always been rice cereal. In Germany, many kids start with carrots or cooked pumpkin. In Holland, they start with bananas or apple mash. There are no studies out there that tell us what the best foods to start with are. Which means that the insistence on cereal in our kids' diet is a tradition, not a necessity. In fact, the AAP has officially stated that we need to "throw out the rice cereal."

When you get right down to it, rice cereal is starch, and sometimes iron-fortified starch. If we are giving it, and it decreases the amounts of breastmilk or formula the child takes, we aren't doing them any favors nutritionally. Our focus should be on good carbohydrates and protein.

Cereals started as an important part of a child's diet back when the infant formula companies couldn't get an absorbable form of iron into the formula. They then fortified rice cereal with iron and introduced the rice cereal early into the diet as a way to make sure the kids got the iron. Now, all the infant formulas are fortified with iron and, of course, breastmilk has an abundant and easily absorbable supply of iron in it, so we really don't need an extra iron source.

At **six to eight months**, it's probably time to give consideration to baby-led feeding/solids/weaning (whatever they call it where you are). Your child should be exhibiting clues that they are ready to take solids before you actually start them in their diet. (Prior to four months of age, your child has a well-developed "tongue-thrust" reflex, which makes spoon-feeding pretty difficult and extremely messy.) If your child turns away from the spoon, spits the food out at you, and, in general, does not seem to be enjoying meals—he isn't ready for the advancement in the diet. This tongue thrust or non-interest in food can exist for longer than six months—meaning, if your child is six months old and is not ready for solids, no worries. It'll come.

If he is ready to eat, then we should start introducing food. Real food, like fruits and vegetables and meat. It can be home prepared foods or baby food. Start on pureed foods and see what happens. We all have a reflex in the back of our throat that doesn't let us swallow something that we have no business trying to swallow. If we were to try to swallow a golf ball, for example, we would make a horrible face and try to throw up.

This "golf ball" reflex is what stops us from going to more textured foods. I'm not going to say that a child has crossed some magic starting line and therefore can swallow thicker foods. It'll be the ability to handle texture that lets us go forward. I take care of some kids I swear can eat steak at six months and some kids who can't handle anything but pureed food at 14 months. It's up to your child how we move through these textures. And that goes for finger foods, too. Whatever texture they can handle is OK to give—if you're not comfortable trying a new texture, don't! Your child never has to eat Cheerios, ever, and they can go to college on pureed foods. We aren't in a hurry. We can get iron now from many sources, the easiest of which is meat. And meat can be pureed if need be, and is found in the thicker foods.

You can start at whichever feeding you want to—whichever feeding your child seems most interested in trying the new food. Let them eat until they are done. No specific amounts are necessary. Breastfeeding mothers may find that the kids won't eat from them, so daddy may be the better person to be feeding solids.

After each new food, you can wait two or three days to see if signs of an allergic reaction, such as diarrhea, rash, or vomiting, occur, but this is not necessary and need only be done if you have a family history of food allergy.

I like holding off on starting juice until about nine months or later (if at all), when you can bribe your child off the bottle by putting the juice in a cup. Plus, juice can cause diarrhea and diaper rash by making the stool very acidic to the skin.

And there's nothing special about store-purchased baby foods—meaning, if you want to make them yourself, go ahead. I think that if I was a better cook, this is the way I'd have done it.

By **eight months to twelve months**, the growth rate of a child slows a bit, so it's not surprising that their appetites slow down a bit now, too. Children in this age group can usually tolerate food with a little more texture.

There is no minimum amount of breastmilk they should be getting. There is no minimum of solid food. There is no minimum of formula. Kids in this age group are really, really good at taking enough calories to grow. They will eat when they are hungry, drink when they are thirsty, and if you guess wrong, you will wear what you chose. If you do this wrong, and they are hungry, they will squawk at you until you get it right. I have never met a kid who will let their parents starve them, at least not without a fight. But they are not growing as fast as they were, so they don't need that many calories. We are trying to teach this generation to respond to hunger cues, not eat simply because the Packers are on or because it's noon. If they are not hungry, they are really not hungry.

DANGER FOODS TO AVOID—HAVE RISK OF CHOKING

- Spoonfuls of peanut butter (the AAP suggests no peanut butter until after one year of age)
- Popcorn
- Nuts
- Raisins
- Grapes
- Uncooked peas
- Celery
- Hard candy
- Whole hot dogs

HOW DO I SWITCH MY CHILD TO COW'S MILK (AFTER AGE ONE)?

There really isn't any magic to this. In fact, it doesn't have to happen at all. If, at a year of age, your nursing relationship with your child is over, just switch over, without worrying about weaning or a slow transition. Even kids who were on soy or other formulas usually do okay with the switch to cow's milk. And if you are nursing (good for you!), there is still plenty of benefits of breastmilk in this age group—there is no cow out there making better milk for your child than you are. There is no need to wean the one-year-old.

Cow's milk is not the perfect food, despite all that we learn, especially here in Wisconsin where I practice. And I see more problems with kids getting too much milk rather than too little. Too much cow's milk (which is more than 20 to 24 ounces a day) can lead to severe iron deficiency. Iron deficiency in a growing brain is not a good idea, in fact, childhood iron deficiency can cause developmental problems that the kids may not overcome. See, cow's milk has no iron in it. It can interfere with iron absorption and cause a low grade blood loss in some kids by creating an inflammation in the gut. Meat is the best source of iron. Other foods that are fortified with iron have a form that is a little harder to absorb.

The kind of milk you transition to makes little difference to me. Kids need a source of fat in their diet for the first two years of life because the fat helps with brain maturation and development. The AAP had previously said to use whole milk as a way to provide that fat, but there isn't anything special in the fat of whole cow's milk that helps human brains grow. The recommendation now is that two percent or lower fat concentration in milk should be used in children with a family history of a risk factor for heart disease. That pretty much means almost every kid in America. Therefore, unless you come from a very rare family, you do not need whole cow's milk. So...try to make sure your child gets about 30 percent of their calories from fat every day, just like we, as adults, are supposed to do.

I'm Ready to Wean, So How Do I Do It?

As I mentioned before, weaning is one of those decisions that's often accompanied by a twinge of guilt and some regret. I hope you've celebrated every step of this breastfeeding journey, and congratulated yourself for what you have accomplished!

Kids who are ready to wean are distractible, spend less time during feedings, and may be more interested in solid foods. If we let the baby lead in weaning, we wait until they decide they want to nurse, without initiating or refusing to nurse. That way, the baby can cut back on the amount of feedings.

More likely, it's mom who wants, or needs, to wean. There are many ways to do this. The most common involves cutting back on one feeding every three days or so. The feeding should be replaced with lots of cuddling and close contact, and if the baby reacts poorly (they may do things to get more attention), then we should slow down the process. And it's nice to try to replace the "work" feedings first, meaning eliminate the feedings where you will be working or away from the baby first, and leave the nighttime and first morning feedings for last. In fact, you can keep those feedings for months after you eliminate the other ones.

If your breasts get uncomfortable, then pump just enough to relieve the pain. Weaning too quickly can lead to mastitis and plugged ducts. You can use ice packs, acetaminophen, ibuprofen, and cabbage leaves, just as we did during the early days of engorgement. Never do any breast binding—that still shows up as a way to stop milk production in some older references. It can lead to all sorts of bad things!

We should wean the baby to formula if they are under one year of age, and to cow's milk if they are over a year. I don't care which formula or which kind of milk. They can be weaned right to a cup if they are over six months or so.

There are a few things for mom to be aware of. You may need to cut back on the calories you consume now in order to avoid gaining weight. Your breast may be a little, well, saggy for a few months (but they were going to get that way anyway because we know that pregnancy is the cause of the breast changes you experience, not breastfeeding), and you may have milk secretion for several months after you are finished weaning. Your period should start coming back, if it hasn't already, and it may be a bit irregular for a while.

CHAPTER 16.
BABY ISSUES — VITAMIN D SUPPLEMENTS

Vitamin D: Why Do We Need It and How Do We Get It?

This is one of my favorite topics because there are so few times I read research and think, "*Of course that's the answer.*" Too much of what research is about just leads to further questions, which is great—we should always be in pursuit of new knowledge. But sometimes it's nice just to have something "click" and feel like why on earth didn't we think of this before? That sums up the research on Vitamin D supplementation for me. (And, hopefully, explains why this topic gets such a large section: Yes, I think it's that important!)

A few caveats before we start. I am writing from Franklin, Wisconsin, a lovely suburb of Milwaukee, in the United States. Wisconsin is known for cows, cheese, and great football. In fact, Wisconsin's Green Bay Packers famously play on "The Frozen Tundra." We don't get a lot of useful sunshine where I am. I got in a lovely discussion about the necessity of vitamin D supplementation with a reader when I realized that her words were spelled funny—like "coloured." She was in New Zealand. New Zealand is not known for its Frozen Tundra. So I'm writing primarily for those of you living north of Atlanta, the area most at risk for being deficient in Vitamin D.

My experience with vitamin D had been "it's fat soluble, don't take too much" and "strong bones and teeth." Then, the American Academy of Pediatrics recommended that breastfed infants receive supplementary vitamin D. Those recommendations have changed over time to include all children, regardless of mode of feeding, but at the time I was like "what?" and decided to ignore it. How could anything be wrong with breastmilk and why just pick on the breastfed population? As if we didn't have enough obstacles to hurdle to get mothers to breastfeed—now we have this assertion that it's deficient in vitamin D? Phooey.

Yes, I was wrong. I did my homework, read the research, and there's just too much of it to ignore now. We are, in my part of the world, all likely to be insufficient in vitamin D. And for infants, the mode of feeding doesn't matter. All children need at least 400 IU from the first few days of life onwards. If formula-fed, a child would need to take 34 ounces a day to get that amount. It isn't just a breastfed infant issue. (It didn't hurt my acceptance of these recommendations, I admit, when we found out that it was a population problem and not just one where we pick on breastmilk or infants.)

We cannot deny the importance of vitamin D. It's clearly an important part of the immune system for short term and long term issues. We found that children with higher vitamin D amounts are less likely to be hospitalized for RSV. There is an association of low vitamin D levels with lupus; multiple sclerosis; rheumatoid arthritis; diabetes (one and two); colon, breast, and prostate cancer; cardiovascular disease; hypertension; and preterm labor. It probably explains the seasonal variation in influenza. There is probably a link between vitamin D and obesity. I can go on, but it's hard to keep up.

We thought that vitamin D didn't cross into breastmilk, and if it did, it was in low amounts. Of course, if mom is insufficient, so is her milk. Vitamin D crosses just fine when moms have sufficient amounts of vitamin D. One of the first studies I saw (at a presentation given by the author) about supplementing mother/ infant breastfeeding dyads was out of the Medical University of South Carolina. I was struck by how many of the mothers they enrolled were deficient in vitamin D. Now I get it—we're not a sunshine-y state here in Wisconsin. But South Carolina? As a good friend explained: "We like our air conditioning." That's it then, isn't it? We have gone from being outside to being inside. Our lifestyle has changed.

And what about this "it's a fat soluble vitamin—don't take too much" caveat that was drilled into me throughout medical school? Well, problem one: it's not a vitamin, it a hormone. Two: while it may be fat soluble, it's regulated like a hormone, and it takes a ton of it to become dangerous. The reports of vitamin D toxicity involve doses in the hundreds of thousands of international units (IU) over weeks or months.

The best source of vitamin D is the sun. When you get increasing amounts of vitamin D activated by the absorption of ultraviolet radiation from the sun, things like sunscreen and increased melanin pigment (a tan!) make it harder to absorb. People with naturally darker skin, therefore, need more vitamin D. And vitamin D is hard to get from food.

To summarize: Vitamin D is important. It comes from the sun. When there is little sun, we need to supplement. The disagreement is not whether we need it. We disagree on the dose, since as research is done, the dose is constantly changing. Below are some guidelines about the doses.

From the Endocrine Society:

- Infants and children ages 0-1 year require at least 400 IU/day (IU=25 ng) of vitamin D and children one year and older require at least 600 IU/day to maximize bone health. To raise the blood level of vitamin D consistently above 30 ng/ml may require at least 1,000 IU/day of vitamin D.

- Adults aged 19-50 years require at least 600 IU/day of vitamin D to maximize bone health and muscle function, and at least 1,500-2,000 IU/day of vitamin D may be needed to maintain blood level of vitamin D above 30 ng/ml.

- Adults aged 50-70 years and adults older than 70 years require at least 600 IU/day and 800 IU/day, respectively, of vitamin D. At least 1,500-2,000 IU/day of vitamin D may be needed to maintain blood level of vitamin D above 30 ng/ml.

- Pregnant and lactating women require at least 600 IU/day of vitamin D and at least 1,500 IU/day of vitamin D may be needed to maintain blood level of vitamin D above 30 ng/ml.

Doctors Wagner, Taylor, and Hollis, the ones doing many of the studies in lactating and pregnant women, recommend 25-50 IU per kilogram of body weight for children two to 12 years of age. For those weighing more than 50 kg (110 pounds), then 2,000-4,000 IU is recommended. For pregnant women, they recommend 4,000 IU. For lactating women, they suggest 6400 IU a day.

And if it's sunny and the right time of year, at the right latitude, go outside and let Mother Nature take care of things, within reason. We don't need sunburn—we just need a little sun. In my part of the world, that works about three months out of the year. And that may be generous. But boy, do we love it when we can enjoy it!

Of course, one size does not fit all. Talk to your doctor about your circumstances, latitude, and potential risk for vitamin D insufficiency, or consider getting your levels of 25 hydroxy vitamin D {25(OH) D} checked to help with a dose that'll be good for you, and your kids. And have fun watching as the new research keeps coming.

The sun has a purpose. Who knew?

More About Vitamin D Supplementation as It Relates to Infants and Breastfeeding Moms

The American Academy of Pediatrics is now recommending that all children receive vitamin D supplementation to prevent rickets. I've already explained why I think the new research on this is fantastically cool. But guess what? I think the subject is so important that I want to back up a bit and look at Vitamin D itself, then examine how specifically it relates to breastfeeding moms and babies.

So what is vitamin D? Vitamin D isn't really a vitamin. Vitamins cannot be synthesized in the body and, therefore, need to be found in the diet. But vitamin D is formed through interaction of sunlight with skin, so it is better classified as a hormone. It is a hormone necessary for bone strength and growth, and it's a potent immune system modulator. Insufficiency of vitamin D has been associated with a number of auto-immune disorders, including rheumatoid arthritis, multiple sclerosis, and other disorders, as I have mentioned.

Rickets: Vitamin D Deficiency

The deficiency of vitamin D shows up as a bone disease called rickets. We desperately want to prevent the complete deficiency of vitamin D. Rickets was very common in the United States in the early part of the 20th century, with weak bones, seizures, and death being all too common until experiments showed that deficiency of vitamin D was the cause and fortification of milk was started.

Other symptoms of rickets include bowed legs in toddlers, small stature, bone pain, and delayed walking. The disease can be diagnosed with x-rays and blood tests, but can occur before symptoms are visible on a physical examination.

What Are the Risk Factors for Vitamin D Deficiency?

Children can be deficient in vitamin D if they have inadequate stores of it or if they have inadequate exposure to sunlight.

Children who are most likely to have inadequate stores are those who were born prematurely or those born to mothers with low stores of vitamin D (usually because of poor nutrition) at the time of delivery.

The rest of us are in the category of inadequate exposure to sunlight. We aren't in the sun much, especially those of us in colder climates. And when we are in the sun, we are covered by clothes or sunscreen. We should never be exposed to sun without sunscreen, but sunscreens markedly depress vitamin D production in skin. And the darker your skin color, the less vitamin D you make from sunshine.

Why Do We Need a Supplement?

No mammalian milk contains the level of vitamin D that sunlight provides. Cow's milk from the grocery store and formula are fortified with vitamin D.

Breastmilk has a very specific recipe, designed over many hundreds of millions of years to provide exactly what nutrients, vitamins, and infection protection infants need. Breastmilk was never expected to provide more than a slight supplement to the sun. So adequate sunshine is necessary to complement breastfeeding.

But we should be avoiding direct sunlight exposure because of the risk of skin cancer. Since the rates of exclusive breastfeeding for longer periods of time have risen in the United States, the CDC has confirmed more cases of rickets. Rickets can be prevented with vitamin D supplements.

DOES THAT MEAN THERE IS SOMETHING WRONG WITH BREASTMILK?

The vitamin D problem we are addressing is not a breastmilk problem, it is a sunlight exposure problem. This recommendation affects mostly breastfed children because formula and cow's milk are already fortified with vitamin D. And breastfed children are not the only ones at risk. All of us in a climate that lacks sunshine are at risk of vitamin D deficiency.

Recommendations for Supplementation

Universal supplementation of all infants with vitamin D is safe and of proven effectiveness.

All children should receive 400 units daily, an amount found in over-the-counter liquid multivitamins, starting at birth.

Children and adolescents who do not take at least 17 ounces of vitamin D fortified milk daily should also receive a supplement.

Supplementation should continue through childhood and adolescence, and continue over the lifespan unless you are lucky enough to live someplace where sunshine is plentiful.

DON'T WANT TO GIVE YOUR BREASTFEEDING BABY THE VITAMINS BECAUSE THEY TASTE LIKE VOMIT?

Yes, I said vomit. But that's not fair. Some of the preparations available now are better tasting, contain just vitamin D, and are starting to be more accessible, especially through online retailers.

Fantastically cool research is coming out that supplementing mom will help both mom and baby achieve normal Vitamin D levels. What is in dispute is not that we need vitamin D, but how much and from where. We'll be seeing frequent changes in dosing recommendations as more research is published. We are likely to see more recommendations for lactating mothers and pregnant women soon. My opinion is strongly in favor of supplementing the nursing mom (and even those not nursing.) Tablets with 1000 IUs can be found over-the-counter—I just found them at Sam's Club and Pick n Save, and I wasn't even looking that hard!

PART 3.
ADVOCATING FOR OTHER MOMS

CHAPTER 17.
ADVOCATING FOR OTHER BREASTFEEDING MOMS

Surviving the Temple of Doom (Poison Darts, Crumbling Floor, and Giant Boulders)—Breastfeeding in America

There is the great part in the beginning of "Raiders of the Lost Ark" where Indiana Jones finally navigates the passageway to the gold idol he wants, and for one second, he has the idol. There's a glimmer of joy in his eye, and then, well, it all goes to hell. As he runs out, he's attacked and chased by all manner of danger, and when he finally escapes, there's somebody there to tell him how dumb he was to try it in the first place. Yup, breastfeeding in America.

What is Breastfeeding Doom? For starters, I think we have taken away the birth experience from women, and placed it in the hands of experts. I see women taking that back, but slowly. I'm really not an expert there, so I'll leave it at that, but this surrendering of maternal instinct starts early in the birth process.

So you decide to breastfeed. Cool. We've been preaching "Breast is Best" (a slogan that needs to die, but that's another soap box) and you listened. Then what? Well, we make it nearly impossible for you to be successful. We give you the information and make it nearly impossible for you to use it. We set you up to fail.

And being mothers, well, you internalize that failure instead of seeing it for what it is—our fault. The failure and the guilt is the fault of every healthcare professional who didn't know enough to help (or get out of the way!), every employer that didn't help with your transition back to work or who provided a short maternity leave, every legislator that voted against the measure to help you get your expenses reimbursed or who felt that breastfeeding in public was something obscene.

I started giving out the t-shirts at one year of age to anybody who breastfed for a year. Why? Well, for some of you it turned out to be an incentive, for others, it was simply a recognition that you survived everything we threw in your way. I love showing you all off.

I am also proud of those of you who tried and met your goals, even if it wasn't a year. And I ache for those of you who wanted a different experience and got swallowed up in the Doom. You shouldn't feel guilty. You should be mad, and I hope you use that energy to change the world.

My to-do list:

1. Talk to legislators.

2010 was a good year for me in Wisconsin in this regard. Our "Right to Breastfeed" bill passed and the federal government passed legislation for workplace support. Now we need to know how those laws are going to be enforced. It's one thing to have the laws—enforcement has yet to be addressed.

We are and need to continue to address truth in advertising and eliminate conflicts of interest.

But it's not all "to-do." Some is already "to celebrate." We are making great progress on providing insurance coverage for breast pumps and for lactation services. Insurance notwithstanding, you can now use your pre-tax dollars for breast pumps. Now that's a victory! We have altered the Federal Tax Code! And we now have federal laws protecting breastfeeding mothers in the workplace.

Some days I feel momentum changing and it feels good. Yes, there's still work and education to be done from a legislative perspective, but we have things to celebrate.

2. Talk to medical professionals.

In case you haven't noticed, I do a ton of this, and I want to do more. I want medical professionals to help, know their limits, or just get out of the way. Hospital cultures need to change and hospital policies need to stop messing up the birth and breastfeeding process and return it to moms and babies. First do no harm, everybody.

3. Make sure that those getting out of the hospital can get, and feel empowered to ask for, help.

I want moms to know that there are tons of people who want to help, and that as a new mom they should ask. I feel sick each time someone says, "I didn't know" or "I didn't want to bother you." Bother me? Bother me? Holy crow. How did that get so messed up? Your medical professionals are working for you. You have the power to find help and encouragement if you need it.

4. Help kids learn that breastfeeding is normal.

That way they grow up knowing that breasts don't just sell burgers and cars.

5. Heal the divide.

This isn't about breastfeeding versus bottlefeeding. This is about the Temple of Doom. The Temple of Doom needs to be overrun, so every mom and baby get a fair chance to be successful.

BREASTFEEDING "STUDIES" AND HOW TO UNDERSTAND THEM

When it comes to healing the divide, I have to say I've noticed that so much of the debate, the passion, the divide itself, comes from "studies" reported in the media about breastfeeding and formula...studies that show which feeding choice is "best," which produces the brightest children, you know that story. And, when it comes to these, I've realized that too many of my patients—and even some of my fellow healthcare providers—read these stories without the critical eye that is so essential when evaluating research.

And so, as a public service to help you as you help me to fight the breastfeeding Temple of Doom, I'm offering this primer on HOW to evaluate research and how to read and understand these studies that so many of us love to quote, or argue against, without even knowing what they mean.

I also offer this information because I have heard from so many breastfeeding moms that the providers with whom they have worked have responded to "evidence" ...meaning studies, policy statement, protocols, etc. So I embark on this subject also considering how it relates to ways you, as a mom, can change the way your healthcare provider practices. I'm going to start with what kind of evidence may be the most persuasive.

I start with information from the United States Preventive Services Task Force (USPSTF). The USPSTF is an independent panel of non-federal experts in prevention and evidence-based medicine and is composed of primary care providers (such as internists, pediatricians, family physicians, gynecologists/obstetricians, nurses, and health behavior specialists). The USPSTF conducts scientific evidence reviews of a broad range of clinical preventive healthcare services (such as screening, counseling, and preventive medications) and develops recommendations for primary care clinicians and health systems. These recommendations are published in the form of "Recommendation Statements." Here's what you need to understand. The USPSTF uses this "quality of evidence" ranking. So we need to as well. It looks like this:

QUALITY OF EVIDENCE

I. Evidence obtained from at least one properly randomized controlled trial.

II. Evidence obtained from well-designed controlled trials without randomization.

III. Evidence obtained from well-designed cohort or case-control analytic studies, preferably from more than one center or research group.

IV. Evidence obtained from multiple time series with or without the intervention. Dramatic results in uncontrolled experiments (such as the results of the introduction of penicillin treatment in the 1940s) could also be regarded as this type of evidence.

V. Opinions of respected authorities, based on clinical experience descriptive studies and case reports, or reports of expert committees.

I'll tackle (I) here—the randomized, controlled trial—the "gold standard" for evaluating treatment or preventive interventions.

All research starts with a question. In the study "The effect of high-dose vitamin D supplementation on serum Vitamin D levels and milk calcium concentration in lactating women and their infants" (Basile et al., 2006), the research question is: "Is high-dose vitamin D effective in increasing 25(OH)D levels in fully breastfeeding mothers to optimal levels without evidence of toxicity?"

The researchers answered this question with a randomized controlled study. This type of study has an intervention (high-dose vitamin D supplementation) and an outcome to measure (serum vitamin D levels). In fact, this study is the best of the best—it's randomized, doubled-blinded, and prospective.

First, subjects are recruited, and then randomized or put into experimental groups based on nothing but chance. This helps eliminate any biases that may be introduced if we got to pick who was put into each experimental group. If we got to pick, we could sway the results in our favor.

The subject is randomly assigned to either the intervention group (the one who gets vitamin D) or the control group (the group that gets nothing or a placebo). In this study, they randomized groups to receive 2000 IU or 4000 IU of vitamin D and had the mothers be their own control group. Then you measure a baseline for the study, like a baseline vitamin D level. In this study, the mothers could be their own controls; after the intervention (taking the vitamin D), they were compared to themselves at baseline before they took the vitamin D. Slick.

Then they took the Vitamin D, and their blood levels were measured, and the authors drew their conclusions.

So, for a randomized controlled trial you get participants, randomize them, do something to one group, then figure out what happened to the group you did something to. If you can find these types of studies, they would be the most persuasive for those needing to be persuaded.

Of course, it's not as easy as this. There are so many other factors to consider when looking at scientific studies and their actual impact on how physicians practice. But for the your sake, and how you might approach a study you want to share with your healthcare provider, let's look next at where your information is coming from.

COMPETENCE, MATH, THE MEDIA, AND MY FAITH IN THE BREASTFEEDING MOTHER

Let's consider this—are you using (or asking your healthcare provider to use) an actual study, or a *report* of a study? Because I have to tell you, if you're bringing information to your healthcare provider to ask him or her to consider it, a *report* of a study just isn't going to do the trick.

I have said before that before we share the media coverage of the study, we should look at the study. Just as an example, let's consider a study about how people perceive breastfeeding mothers. I want us to carefully examine both what the study itself actually said and how the study's findings were reported. See why that's a two-pronged question? In the case of the study we'll examine here, the media coverage was especially inflammatory, so I think it's even more important to go to the source. This one was reported like this: Breastfeeding mothers are seen as incompetent, people don't want to work with them, and they need to be warned about those perceptions.

The study itself is called *"Spoiled Milk: An Experimental Examination of Bias Against Mothers Who Breastfeed"* (Smith, Hawkins, Paull, 2011). The title is telling. The word choice is significant—"spoiled" and "bias against" show right up front that we aren't looking for happy endings.

The authors state in the abstract that they are "drawing from the objectification literature" and that they are testing "the hypothesis that breastfeeding mothers are the victims of bias." Victims.

"Objectification" means that people are looking at body parts as "things" that are then used or looked at by other people. Breasts fall into this category.

The authors also contend that reproduction, including menstruation, pregnancy, and lactation is "devalued" and "serve as cues that women are inferior." I checked out their cited sources. None mentioned lactation. Later, they agree, and they themselves say that the "research on perception of breastfeeding is sparse." They go on to cite one study that did look at perception of breastfeeding which showed that the "woman who breastfed was rated positively, including being a good mother, and as highly feminine." They question this study because they question whether those surveyed just gave the answer they thought was right. I think, based on this, that their mentioning lactation as being devalued was not based on the research. They do a good job of showing how menstruating women are exposed to bias. And that bias takes the form of being seen as less competent.

So, they start with two hypotheses: One I said was objectification; the second is "paternalistic prejudice."

With objectification, they hypothesize that breastfeeding mothers will be seen as having lower levels of competence and "warmth." Paternalistic prejudice, which sees mothers as less competent, also sees them as having more "warmth." So, the authors hypothesize two possible outcomes: Breastfeeding mothers will be seen as less competent, and they will either be seen as being warm or not. If their experiments show breastfeeding mothers to be warm, but less competent, that will be proof of paternalistic prejudice. If they are both warm and less competent, the bias breastfeeding mothers are exposed to is objectification. They will find a bias though, it seems.

There is a lot of discussion of the objectification of the breast, and they use the recent Facebook events to prove their point. As if they needed Facebook to prove that Americans objectify breasts. Interestingly, they talk about how a woman's perceptions of herself as an object will contribute to her feelings about breastfeeding in public, with women who see themselves more as objects feeling more shame and embarrassment. Of course, this isn't what the study was addressing. Bummer.

The study also mentions that breastfeeding can remind people of the "animalistic nature of humanity" and that is threatening to some, leading to less favorable ratings of breastfeeding mothers. I haven't yet pulled that study. I doubt I could. And they mention that other studies showing that if a person is uncomfortable with anything sexual they rated breastfeeding women as less favorable.

So, in their introduction, I see lots of words chosen to evoke negative emotion. I see a set-up that Western society's objectification of breasts is the problem. And I find it interesting, and an opportunity to help a mother who feels this way, that feeling as if you are an object impacts your breastfeeding experience without anyone else messing it up for you. The authors don't do a good job of separating individual self-perception with public perception.

Okay, the actual experiments:

In the first one, 30 students with a mean age of 19 years, who are 83 percent white, are asked to evaluate a celebrity under a guise of a class project. They chose Brooke Shields as the celebrity. They gave the participants her resume and included information that she was going to write a book. One group was told that the book would contain her experiences with bottle-feeding, the other with breastfeeding. They rated eight general competence traits and seven general warmth traits. Math skills were included to assess competence in a gender-stereotyped subject. We are hearing a bunch about this math thing in the media, aren't we? It was a measure of performance in a man-associated skill.

The result? High warmth. Low competence. So, paternalistic prejudice. But, was this really all about breastfeeding? Maybe it was about Brooke. Maybe it was about not wanting to do an assignment like this when you are 19.

In the second study, they wanted to know whether the study participants would rate themselves as less competent in math (man stuff) if they were a breastfeeding woman, a woman with sexualized breasts, or a woman with non-sexualized breasts.

This study started with 65 participants, but four were dropped because they had kids. The remaining 61 percent were 68 percent female, 92 percent white, and about 20 years old. Let me just say, one of the neat things about a good study is that it is "generalizable" to the general population. This one—not so much.

They asked them about an ad for nipple cream for "chaffed nipples after"... nursing, exercise, or to "refresh nipples" before intimacy. The woman they used in the ad was wearing a sweatshirt. Apparently, a non-sexy one.

Results? No difference on "warmth." Decreased general competence. Decreased workplace competence (uhm...was this part of the hypothesis?) No difference in math. No measure of girl skills (which they say is verbal skills). No control group. That means...useless results. Of course, they didn't say that.

The third study, the participants are again young, white, and childless. And I'm so confused by what they do here, I don't even want to go into it. In fact, I'm bored.

They say the results for study three showed no change in warmth and less competence. I have to take their word for it because it is dense material. So, study one equals paternalistic prejudice. Study two showed nothing. Study three showed low competence and no change in warmth, which doesn't fit into their paradigm. Their conclusions include this statement: *"We can only speculate that the evidence for bias would be magnified if people were to rate an actual woman engaging in public nursing."* Emphasis mine. I put it in italics since I can't gag on it in print form.

I don't think they proved anything. People who think breasts are for sex wouldn't like breastfeeding—check. College students don't think breastfeeding mothers have good man-type skills. Check. I'm just going to put this out there—college students are exploring, questioning, gaining independence, and finding out who they are, including sexually. Maybe they aren't perfect for defining the role of breastfeeding in the workplace.

What was interesting was all the self-perception data. If we can convince a mother to have more confidence in herself, to value who she is, that makes a difference. But we knew that confidence in your own self-worth, your own body is what can make or break a breastfeeding relationship. That was the lesson of this study. They missed it. We shouldn't.

"Breastfeeding and Child Behavior in the Millennium Cohort Study." What Does It Mean?

For my last example, this time looking most specifically at what a study actually *means,* I'll refer to the particular study (Heikkilä et al., 2011) described above, which concludes that in "singleton, white UK children, breastfeeding for four months or longer was associated with lower odds of behavioral problems at five years."

I read it. The authors didn't make claims that weren't in the study. They ignored the right data, since it was invalid statistically. They separated exclusive from partial breastfed children. They discounted the preterm infant data since it was statistically no good. Looks good.

Now, what good did it do? *shrug*

Can we generalize it to the population? Well, the white kids in the UK, certainly. Other ethnic groups didn't turn in the tool the authors were using to measure behavior. That seems more interesting to me, but if you don't have the data, you don't have the data.

Do these studies ("Breastfeeding makes boys smarter, but not girls," "Breastfeeding helps improve lower extremity muscle strength," "Breastfeeding for four months makes a better – behaved white kindergartner") help?

And how about those "guilt" rebuttals? When we size up the positive results from the study with the negative press from it, we need to start talking about how to handle the backlash. What language do we use? See why these are all important questions? And so I ask you to consider them carefully, both when discussing a study in general, and more specifically when bringing it to your healthcare provider and asking for specific action (or reaction) based on it.

And that leads me to my last step of advocacy (or perhaps it should be the first?)...what to do when the person you relied upon for breastfeeding information instead gave you bad advice.

A Pediatrician's Plea to Breastfeeding Mothers: Did You Get Bad Info? Please Speak UP!

Too often, new families get unsupportive or uninformed breastfeeding care from their providers. Systems of healthcare vary around the world, but the lack of breastfeeding education doesn't seem to be confined to any one profession, country, and type of healthcare delivery system or model of care. I'm going to stick with American allopathic medical care, and probably pediatrics in general, since that's what I am and what I know.

And what I know, as I have said before, is this: We have given much of the power of parenting away to "experts." My wish is for mothers to take that power back and to feel confident enough to speak up. I know that the responsibility of listening should rest with the provider, and ideally, the mother should not have to struggle to make herself heard. But it seems as if maybe that doesn't always happen (she writes, facetiously).

I acknowledge that physicians, pediatricians especially, should absolutely know something about breastfeeding, and if they don't, they should do something to remedy that or at the very least, find someone to whom to refer. But meanwhile, the truth is that we have a while to wait and work before that happens. The information is out there, as is the help. Getting the resources to the provider and having them pay attention to the resources is the stumbling block. I'm convinced the key to getting providers to pay attention lies with you and with all mothers.

Here's the thing, again, as I have said before: Healthcare providers are the hired help. We are the people that a family has chosen to help them through their journey. We are supposed to give the information they need to make an informed decision, to help aid in the encouragement of and confidence in parenting choices. If we don't have that info, we aren't doing our job.

But we are responsible for lots of information. We need to learn that infant feeding is a priority in the knowledge base for the families that have entrusted their care to us. Lots of agencies and organizations are working to help providers see that infant feeding is an absolute priority and the provision of excellent care.

But we need to have that reinforced by our patients. Does it stink that mothers need to speak up despite the fact that nearly 80 percent of new mothers choose to breastfeed? Yes, of course. Yes, yes, yes. Do we need mothers to help? YES! Help.

How can you help? Simply by speaking up, even though that shouldn't necessarily be your "job." Bring good studies to your healthcare providers and ask them to consider them. Let them know when you feel you've received bad advice. Because, yes, I've been thinking a lot about what mothers can do when they get unsupportive or uninformed breastfeeding care from their doctors. I've heard from so many breastfeeding moms about providers who tell them to wean or pump and dump unnecessarily, who state that breastfeeding has no value after a few months, who blame all dental problems on breastfeeding...the list goes on and on.

I'm sorry about this. I wish I could change it, magically, overnight, so no mom ever had to experience it again. But, of course, that is not going to happen. And so we all have to change it together, one step at a time. I hope you're ready to start making those steps with me, changing our little corners of the world as best we can.

In other words, I ask you to please speak up. And some day, hopefully, we can all celebrate the good advice and support breastfeeding moms receive. Which is how I'd like to end this look at abolishing the Breastfeeding Temple of Doom, by examining it in terms of a lifelong cycle, rather than a fragmented journey.

AND SO I ASK: WHO IS YOUR BREASTFEEDING SPECIALIST?

Whenever I talk to new parents, I love to remind them to celebrate the journey, to place the discussion in the now and not in what the might be. Each step in their child's life is special and finite. As a pediatrician, I am dedicated to the health of children, hopefully sending them on their way to being healthy adults. And I know that a healthy little girl who becomes a healthy adolescent, and eventually a mother, has better pregnancy outcomes and has healthy babies. I love being a lactation consultant because I get to watch all parts of that cycle.

The journey is so fragmented, though. Discontinuity marks the transition from womb to breast, from fetus to newborn, from pregnancy to motherhood. We fragment and compartmentalize hospital to outpatient care, from new mom to working mom, and the role of wife and mother. We separate babes and mothers, separate instinct from societal expectation, and transfer care among providers, buildings, and philosophies. And we have somehow lost our continuity of wisdom from generation to generation.

Someday, we will collaborate and coordinate. We will appreciate that healthy babies will grow to be healthy mothers who will give birth to healthy babies, and we will celebrate that cycle. I'm hoping some day we don't have an individual person to point to when we ask, "Who can help me breastfeed?" That hospitals, providers, daycares, employers, family support systems, shopping centers, and lawmakers will all know what their roles are, and we will clear our obstacles to breastfeeding success.

Someday, when we ask, *"Who is your breastfeeding specialist?"* the answer will be, *"We all can help."*

EPILOGUE:
EVERYTHING YOU NEED TO KNOW
TO BE A PERFECT PARENT

Catchy title, huh? C'mon, you've bought books with titles like this. Maybe they're even next to your bed, along with a stack of pregnancy books that implied that if you looked the wrong way at a fish your kid would have three arms.

I find that most of the phone calls I get from tearful, overwhelmed families are almost always because a book they are reading is telling them their child isn't doing something they should be doing. And because the child isn't following the book, something terrible must be happening and they suck as parents.

These are the books that tell you kids can be potty trained in a day, that four-month-olds can "soothe" themselves, that you can train a baby to conform to your schedule...the books I hope all of you will close, put on a shelf, or throw away because of the stress and sense of failure they induce.

Perfect parenting means making mistakes.

OK. Maybe "making mistakes" is too harsh. How about "learning by trial and error." My husband is a psychiatrist, and between the two of us, you'd think we'd have enough training to get the parenting of our three boys just about right. But even we have learned that you need to change a little boy's diaper with your mouth closed, that disciplining without laughing is key, and that our boys are people, with personalities, who have schedules and needs that sometimes are not the same as ours. We're better parents because we have learned from our errors. Or maybe, it's not an error, it's an experience. We have tried something, it didn't work, and we've moved on despite what a book, theory, or adamently-stated alternative opinion suggested.

It takes an empowered parent to ignore a barrage of advice. We need to work on empowerment, and reclaim our parenting instincts. We give too many of them away. I am confused and saddened by how strongly some parents feel that what they are doing is right and that all people need to follow what they did because it worked for them. We have many experts in our lives, all with different qualifications and powers of persuasion. Here's the thing about those expert opinions, health recommendations, and studies: They are meant for a population and can be individualized. The reverse is not true. What may be true for an individual or a family cannot and should not be extrapolated to a general health recommendation. We do that all too often. Just like the books that promise everything, we have to realize that all of us will have different parenting experiences. While it's wonderful to share what has worked and not worked for us, hopefully, we don't send our advice out as a public health recommendation.

Realistically, there are very few absolutes in parenting, and I'm a passionate believer in parental intuition and instinct. With few exceptions, doing whatever works best for your family, even if it means some trial and error, is the way to become a "perfect parent."

APPENDIX

First Week Daily Breastfeeding Log

How The Log Works

Answer These Questions on Day 4, 5, or 6

Resources

FIRST WEEK DAILY BREASTFEEDING LOG

Call us if you do not meet the number in the Goal column

Breastfeeding warm line: 262-687-2756 or Dr. Jenny Rucka Thomas: 262-687-6620

DAY 1   GOAL

Hour of Feeding	12 1 2 3 4 5 6 7 8 9 10 11 12 1 2 3 4 5 6 7 8 9 10 11	8
Wet Diaper	One	1
Black Tarry Stool	One	1

DAY 2   GOAL

Hour of Feeding	12 1 2 3 4 5 6 7 8 9 10 11 12 1 2 3 4 5 6 7 8 9 10 11	8
Wet Diaper	One Two	2
Dark Brown Stool	One Two	2

DAY 3   GOAL

Hour of Feeding	12 1 2 3 4 5 6 7 8 9 10 11 12 1 2 3 4 5 6 7 8 9 10 11	8
Wet Diaper	One Two Three	3
Dark Green Stool	One Two Three	3

DAY 4   GOAL

Hour of Feeding	12 1 2 3 4 5 6 7 8 9 10 11 12 1 2 3 4 5 6 7 8 9 10 11	8
Wet Diaper	One Two Three Four	4
Green-Yellow Stool	One Two Three Four	4

Day 5   **Goal**

Hour of Feeding	12 1 2 3 4 5 6 7 8 9 10 11 12 1 2 3 4 5 6 7 8 9 10 11	8
Wet Diaper	One Two Three Four Five	5
Yellow Stool	One Two Three Four	4

Day 6   **Goal**

Hour of Feeding	12 1 2 3 4 5 6 7 8 9 10 11 12 1 2 3 4 5 6 7 8 9 10 11	8
Wet Diaper	One Two Three Four Five Six	6
Yellow Stool	One Two Three Four	4

Day 7   **Goal**

Hour of Feeding	12 1 2 3 4 5 6 7 8 9 10 11 12 1 2 3 4 5 6 7 8 9 10 11	8
Wet Diaper	One Two Three Four Five Six	6
Yellow Stool	One Two Three Four	4

How the Log Works

This chart is for your first, often difficult, week of nursing. **You need to call** if you don't meet the number in the GOAL column.

Day 1 is the first 24 hours of your new baby's life. **Day 2** is the second 24 hours, and so on.

The numbers across the top are the hours in the day. You'll notice that there isn't any place to chart how long the baby fed on each breast. That was done on purpose. *It isn't the length of time, but the quality of the feeding that counts.* My son and I both have a bowl of Cocoa Puffs every morning, the same amount, in the same size bowl. It takes him like 20 minutes to finish off the bowl, whereas I inhale it in about 45 seconds. It's the same bowl of Cocoa Puffs.

The goal of eight feedings is so that mom gets stimulation on her breasts every three hours. I think we talk out of both sides of our mouths as medical professionals—we tell you to feed "on demand" and then say make sure the baby eats every three hours. The "every three hours" is important because we are trying to get mom's level of prolactin, the hormone that makes milk, up to levels where she can sustain lactation for as long as she chooses. Prolactin is stimulated by suckling at the breast and the level starts to fall after about three hours. The level of prolactin starts to plateau after about two to three weeks, so we can let the baby and mom go a little longer between feedings then.

Since we don't care how long the baby stays on, and we want to make sure that mom's nipples get stimulated every three hours, you just have to check off the hour in which the baby feeds, making sure baby gets eight feedings a day.

Wet diapers—pretty self-explanatory. You should see one wet diaper on day 1, two on day 2, three on day 3, up to about six on day 6 and after.

Stools—This column tells you the color and amount to expect each day. The stool needs to be bigger than a 50 cent piece in order to count. We should have yellow stool on day 4 if all's going well.

ANSWER THESE QUESTIONS ON DAY 4, 5, OR 6

Please call us if you circle any answers in the Right hand column.

Breastfeeding baby warm line: 262-687-2756 or Dr. Jenny Rucka Thomas: 262-687-6220

Do you feel breastfeeding is going well?	Yes	No
Has your milk come in yet? Did your breasts feel firm or full between days 2 and 4 after delivery?	Yes	No
Do your breasts feel full before feedings and/or empty after feeding?	Yes	No
Are your nipples extremely sore? Do you dread feedings?	No	Yes
Do you experience pain with feedings?	No	Yes
Is your baby able to latch on to your breasts? (Opens wide and gets about ½ inch behind the nipple into his/her mouth)	Yes	No
Does your baby ask to feed? (Answer no if you have to wake the baby most of the time)	Yes	No
Does your baby nurse about every 2-3 hours, at least 8 times in 24 hours?	Yes	No
Is your baby having yellow seedy bowel movements?	Yes	No
Does your baby seem hungry after feedings? (crying, fussy, sucking hands)	No	Yes
Is your baby wetting his/her diapers at least 4-6 times in 24 hours?	Yes	No

Resources

Websites Mentioned in the Book:

Business Case for Breastfeeding: www.ask.hrsa.gov

Dr. Hale's study on Candida (yeast): www.ncbi.nlm.nih.gov/pubmed/19500049

Hand Expression: http://newborns.stanford.edu/Breastfeeding/HandExpression.html

Human Milk Banking Association of North America (HMBANA): www.HMBANA.org

Infant Risk Center: www.infantrisk.com

Medications to Increase Milk Supply: www.breastfeedingonline.org

WHO Growth Charts: (http://www.cdc.gov/growthcharts/who_charts.htm)

Helpful Websites:

Baby-led breastfeeding: http://www.geddesproduction.com/breast-feeding-baby-led.php

Biological Nurturing: http://www.biologicalnurturing.com/

Skin-to-skin: http://massbreastfeeding.org/index.php/handouts/

Find a lactation consultant: http://www.ilca.org/i4a/pages/index.cfm?pageid=3432

Health professionals' attitudes and use of nipple shields for breastfeeding women: http://www.ncbi.nlm.nih.gov/pubmed/20524842

Nipple shields: a review of the literature. http://www.ncbi.nlm.nih.gov/pubmed/20807104

Chapter 17

Media Coverage of Spoiled Milk Articles:

http://www.bnet.com/blog/health-fit-tips/
how-breastfeeding-can-hurt-careers/574

http://www.sciencenewsline.com/psychology/2011041513000065.html

http://www.citytowninfo.com/career-and-education-news/articles/
breastfeeding-mothers-seen-as-less-competent-study-finds-11042501

http://blogs.wsj.com/ideas-market/2011/04/21/
breastfeeding-women-viewed-as-incompetent/

BIBLIOGRAPHY

Academy of Breastfeeding Medicine Protocol Committee. (2008). ABM clinical protocol #6: Guideline on co-sleeping and breastfeeding. *Breastfeeding Medicine, 3*(1), 38-43. Retrieved from http://www.bfmed.org/Resources/Protocols.aspx.

Academy of Breastfeeding Medicine Protocol Committee. (2010). ABM clinical protocol #22: Guidelines for management of jaundice in the breastfeeding infant equal to or greater than 35 weeks' gestation. Breastfeeding Medicine, 5(2), 87-93. Retrieved from http://www.bfmed.org/Resources/Protocols.aspx.

American Academy of Pediatrics, Section on Breastfeeding. (2005). Breastfeeding and the Use of Human Milk. *Pediatrics, 115*(2), 496-506.

American Academy of Pediatrics. (2009). Safe and healthy beginnings: A resource toolkit for hospitals and physicians' offices. Elk Grove Village, IL: AAP.

Adkins, Y., & Lönnerdal, B. (2003). Potential host-defense role of a human milk vitamin B-12 binding protein, haptocorrin, in the gastrointestinal tract of breastfed infants, as assessed with porcine haptocorrin in vitro. *The American Journal of Clinical Nutrition, 77*(5), 1234-1240.

Basile, L.A., Taylor, S.N., Wagner, C.L., Horst, R.L., & Hollis, B.W. (2006). The effect of high-dose vitamin D supplementation on serum Vitamin D levels and milk calcium concentration in lactating women and their infants. *Breastfeed Med, 1*(1), 27-35.

Bernt KM, & Walker,W.A. (1999). Human milk as a carrier of biochemical messages. *Acta Paediatr Suppl, 88*(430), 27-41.

Biasucci, G., Rubini, M., Riboni, S., Morelli, L., Bessi, E. & Retetangos, C. (2010). Mode of delivery affects the bacterial community in the newborn gut. *Early Human Development, 86*(1, Supplement), 13-15.

Cattaneo, A. (2008). The benefits of breastfeeding or the harm of formula feeding? *Journal of Paediatrics and Child Health, 44*(1-2), 1-2.

Feldman-Winter, L.B., Schanler, R.J., O'Connor, K.G., & Lawrence, R.A. (2008). Pediatricians and the promotion and support of breastfeeding. *Arch Pediatr Adolesc Med, 162*(12), 1142-1149.

Forchielli, M.L. & Walker, W.A. (2005). The role of gut-associated lymphoid tissues and mucosal defence. *British Journal of Nutrition, 93*(SupplementS1), S41-S48.

Gartner, L. (2007). Hyperbilirubinemia and breastfeeding. In Hale, T., & Hartmann, P. (Eds.). Textbook of human lactation. Amarillo, TX: Hale Publishing.

Gatti, L. (2008). Maternal perceptions of insufficient milk supply in breastfeeding. *Journal of Nursing Scholarship, 40*(4), 355-363.

Gettler, L.T., & McKenna, J.J. (2011). Evolutionary perspectives on mother–infant sleep proximity and breastfeeding in a laboratory setting. *American Journal of Physical Anthropology, 144*(3), 454-462.

Gnoth, M.J., Kunz, C., Kinne-Saffran, E. & Rudloff, S. (2000). Human milk oligosaccharides are minimally digested in vitro. *The Journal of Nutrition, 130*(12), 3014-3020.

Grummer-Strawn, L., & Shealy, K. (2009). Progress in protecting, promoting, and supporting breastfeeding: 1984–2009. *Breastfeeding Medicine, 4*(s1), S-31-S-39.

Hall, R.T., Mercer, A.M., Teasley, S.L., McPherson, D.M., Simon, S.D., Meyers, B.M., et al. (2002). A breast-feeding assessment score to evaluate the risk for cessation of breast-feeding by 7 to 10 days of age. *The Journal of Pediatrics, 141*(5), 659-664.

Hanson, L. (2004). *Immobiology of human milk: How breastfeeding protects babies.* Amarillo, Texas: Pharmasoft Publishing.

Heikkilä, K., Sacker, A., Kelly, Y., Renfrew, M.J., Quigley, M.A. (2011). Breast feeding and child behavior in the Millennium Cohort Study. Arch Dis Child, 96(7); 635-642.

Ip, S., Chung, M., Raman, G., Trikalinos, T.A. & Lau, J. (2009). A summary of the Agency for Healthcare Research and Quality's evidence report on breastfeeding in developed countries. *Breastfeeding Medicine, 4*(s1), S-17-S-30.

Kvåle G, & Heuch, I. (1988). Lactation and cancer risk: is there a relation specific to breast cancer? *J Epidemiol Community Health, 42*(1), 30-37.

Lawrence, R.A., & Lawrence, R.M. (2011). *Breastfeeding: A guide for the medical profession,* 7th edition. Maryland Heights, MD: Elsevier.

LeBouder, E., Rey-Nores, J.E., Raby, A.C., Affolter, M., Vidal, K., Thornton, C.A., & Labeta, M.O. (2006). Modulation of neonatal microbial recognition: TLR-mediated innate immune responses are specifically and differentially modulated by human milk. *The Journal of Immunology, 176*(6), 3742-3752.

Nyqvist, K.H., Expert Group of the International Network on Kangaroo Mother Care, Anderson, G.C., Bergman, N., Cattaneo, A., Charpak, N., et al. (2010). State of the art and recommendations. Kangaroo mother care: application in a high-tech environment. *Acta Pædiatrica, 99*(6), 812-819.

Penders, J., Thijs, C., Vink, C., Stelma, F.F., Snijders, B., Kummeling, I., et al. (2006). Factors influencing the composition of the intestinal microbiota in early infancy. *Pediatrics, 118*(2), 511-521.

Shulman R.J., Shanler, R.J., Lau, C., Heitkemper, M.,Ou, C.N., & Smith, E.O. (1998). Early feeding, antenatal glucocorticoids, and human milk decrease intestinal permeability in preterm infants. *Pediatric Research, 44*(4): p. 519-523.

Smith, J.L., Hawkinson, K., Paull, K. (2011). Spoiled milk: An experimental examination of bias against mothers who breastfeed. *Pers Soc Psychol Bull, 37*(7), 867-878.

Subcommittee on Hyperbilirubinemia. (2004). Management of hyperbilirubinemia in the newborn infant 35 or more weeks of gestation. *Pediatrics, 114*(1), 297-316.

U.S. Department of Health and Human Services. (2011). *The Surgeon General's Call to Action to Support Breastfeeding,* Washington, DC: US Department of Health and Human Services, Office of the Surgeon General.

US Preventive Services Task Force, Screening of Infants for Hyperbilirubinemia to Prevent Chronic Bilirubin Encephalopathy. (2009). US Preventive Services Task Force Recommendation Statement. *Pediatrics, 124*(4), 1172-1177.

Wagner C, Taylor, S.N., & Hollis, B.W. (2010). *New insights into vitamin d during pregnancy, lactation and early infancy.* Amarillo, Texas: Hale Publishing, L.P.

Wessel, M.A., Cobb, J.C., Jackson, E.B., Harris, G.S. Jr., & Detwiler, A.C. (1954). Paroxysmal fussing in infancy, sometimes called "colic." *Pediatrics, 14*(5), 421-435.

INDEX

About the Authors

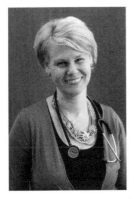

Dr. Jenny Thomas is a noted breastfeeding expert and is among a small handful of practicing pediatricians who are also board-certified lactation consultants (IBCLC). She is a fellow of the Academy of Breastfeeding Medicine; the current Chief of the Chapter Breastfeeding Coordinators for the American Academy of Pediatric's (AAP) Section on Breastfeeding; and the current Chair of the Wisconsin Breastfeeding Coalition. She won an AAP Special Achievement Award in 2009 for her advocacy work, including testifying before the state legislature regarding breastfeeding laws. She has earned her Masters of Public Health degree. She is the mother of three children, all breastfed with varying degrees of success.

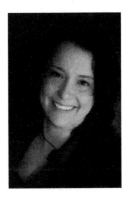

Lisa Holewa is a best-selling book author and an award-winning national news reporter with a special interest in children's issue. She is the co-author of the parenting guide: *What Kindergarten Teachers Know: Practical and Playful Ways for Parents to Help Children Listen, Learn and Cooperate at Home.* She worked for ten years as a reporter for The Associated Press, and her stories have appeared in newspapers world-wide. She is the mother of three children.

Ordering Information

Hale Publishing, L.P.
1712 N. Forest Street
Amarillo, Texas, USA 79106

8:00 am to 5:00 pm CST

Call » 806.376.9900
Toll free » 800.378.1317
Fax » 806.376.9900

Online Orders
www.ibreastfeeding.com